BODYMA1

GW00746483

David Filkin was Editor of BBC television's *Tomorrow's World* from
1979 to 1985, when he became Editor of *QED*, the wide-ranging
BBC 1 science series. During his long and successful television
career he has been responsible for many popular science-related
programmes, of which *Bodymatters* and *Brainstorm* are the most recent.
His previous books include *Tomorrow's World Today* (1984).

DAVID FILKIN

BODYMATTERS

A magical mystery tour of our own flesh and blood

BBC BOOKS

Published by BBC Books,
a division of BBC Enterprises Limited,
Woodlands, 80 Wood Lane, London W12 0TT
First published 1988
© David Filkin 1988
Illustrations © David Cook/Linden Artists 1988
ISBN 0 563 20677 2 (paperback)
ISBN 0 563 20705 1 (hardback)
Set in 9/10 Univers Light by Ace Filmsetting Ltd, Frome
Printed in Great Britain by Cambus Litho, East Kilbride
Bound in Great Britain by Hunter & Foulis Ltd, Edinburgh
Colour separations by Dot Gradations Ltd, Chelmsford
Jacket and cover printed by Fletchers of Norwich

CONTENTS

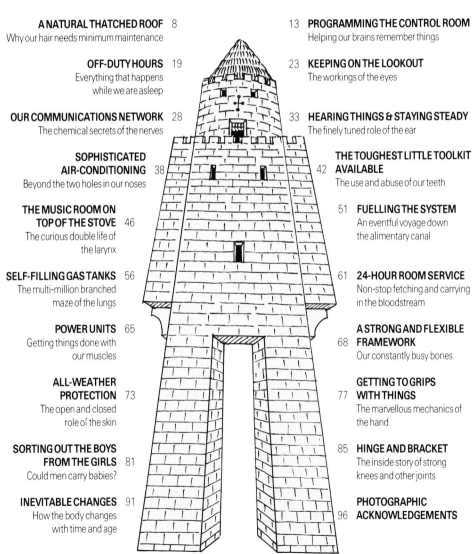

THE LIVING CITADEL

Most of us think of ourselves as one single living thing. But in fact every one of us is much more complex; a unique combination of billions of living cells, all of them busily helping each other to keep the whole community of cells fed and watered, alive and kicking. Our bodies are rather like well-built fortress towns, protecting a busy working population which in turn keeps the citadel impregnable and effective.

Some of our living cells are the building materials from which the citadel is constructed; instead of bricks, stones and mortar we have bone, skin and tissue cells. Deep inside there are other kinds of cells, making miles of wires and pipes; just like the electric cables and plumbing in real buildings. Of course these are the nerves which carry messages between the brain and every other part of us; and the blood vessels through which blood is pumped, dropping off vital supplies all round the body, and picking up the refuse at the same time.

Other living cells are like the people who live in any town: housekeepers and labourers, craftsmen with special skills, managers, politicians, policemen and soldiers. All of them have important jobs; our housekeeping cells, for instance, keep the buildings clean, tidy and properly supplied when everything is working normally. But if disaster strikes and the fabric of the building gets damaged – if we cut or burn ourselves, for instance – then the labouring cells and the craftsmen repair the damage. Our police cells are always on the lookout for invading bacteria and viruses, and our soldiers are marshalled to fight them as soon as they are discovered.

If we could shrink ourselves down, like Alice in Wonderland, to the size of a single living cell, we could explore the intricate workings of our bodies as if we were tourists in some exotic foreign city. The manager and politician cells in our minds can help us to imagine and understand things; and if we get the cells in our eyes to help them, we can easily go on a magical mystery tour of our living citadel through the pages of this book.

7

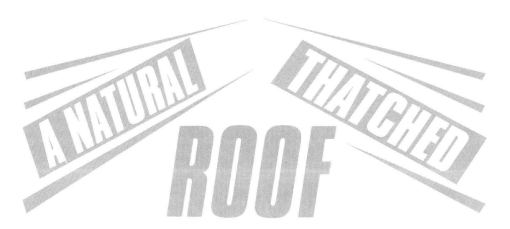

A NATURAL THATCHED ROOF

If we start our tour at the top of the citadel, the first place to explore is the roof. And for most humans it is a thatched roof. When we talk of our hair we nearly always mean the hair on our heads; the natural roof that protects us from sun, rain and injury.

In fact we have hair virtually all over our bodies. Apart from special areas, like our lips, nipples, the palms of our hands and the soles of our feet, the entire surface of our skin is covered with almost invisible hairs. Most of us can see the thicker hairs on top of our arms, say; but hold the underside of your arm up against a strong light, and you will also be able to make out a fine fuzz of hair. The hair on our heads, arms and legs, the more obvious pubic and underarm hair, and this fuzzy hair all provide warmth and protection. Our hairs stand on end when we get goose pimples, trapping a layer of air to insulate us against the cold; they lie flat and retain a cooling film of evaporating perspiration on our skin when we get too hot.

But it is the hair on our heads which everyone notices. And not surprisingly, we tend to show it off in ways that show how we want to be seen. What does a close-shaven head mean to you compared with a long-haired style? For one person, images of skinheads and rockers might come to mind. Someone else might think of American soldiers and hippies. Or astronauts and pop stars. In fact it is very easy to jump to conclusions about people just because of their hairstyles.

In order to send out messages about ourselves, we style our hair with the aid of dyes and chemicals, hot water and gels. But what do all these substances do to its health? When you start finding out about hair, the first surprising fact you discover is that most of it is actually dead. But it's still incredibly strong. (Perhaps you have seen one of those circus acts where an acrobat spins round while dangling from a trapeze to which she is attached only by her hair?) And that strength can be weakened if you mistreat your hair.

Of course we all have different natural hair. Whether we are born with blonde or brunette, straight or curly, thick or fine hair depends on the characteristics we inherit from our parents and grandparents. If you are an Oriental person you will have more head hairs than any other racial type – about 120 000 to be precise, as opposed to 110 000 hairs on the typical Afro-Caribbean head, 100 000 on a Caucasian blonde and a mere 80 000 on the average redhead. But whatever our differences, we all have hair that is structured the same way, with the same life-cycle and development.

All over our skin are tiny pockets called hair follicles. They are a bit like minute flower pots which are specially prepared for the growing of a hair rather than a flower. They need 'switching on', however, before a mature hair can start growing in them. This is done by the male hormone, testosterone, even in females. (That is why, at puberty, when there are a lot of male and female hormones being prod-

uced in our bodies, pubic and underarm hairs start to emerge.)

Once the follicle is 'switched on', nutrients are drawn from the bloodstream into the papilla, a kind of hair root at the bottom of the follicle. There the nutrients are converted into hair cells, which produce a kind of leathery protein to give hair its special strength. As millions and millions of these hair cells are produced, they force their way up the hair follicle, rather like

All our hairs, however long, are rooted in the skin and grow in the same way. The cross-section shows how living cells die off and compact into a strong hair by the time they are pushed up above the skin's surface.

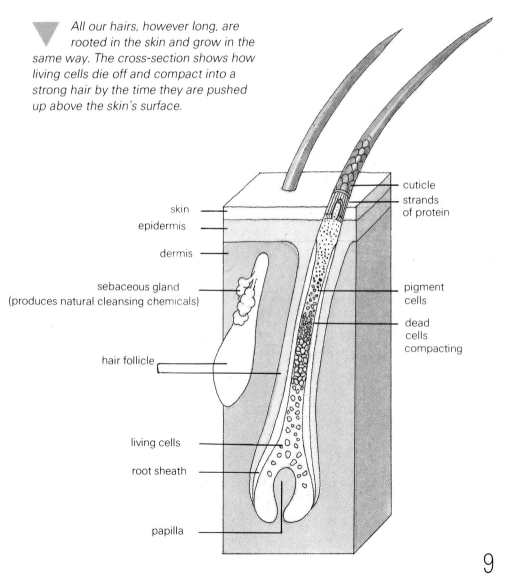

skin
epidermis
dermis
sebaceous gland
(produces natural cleansing chemicals)
hair follicle
living cells
root sheath
papilla

cuticle
strands
of protein

pigment
cells

dead
cells
compacting

9

toothpaste being squeezed up a tube. On the way they also get mixed up with pigment cells, which give the hair its colour. (As some people grow older, the pigment cells stop being produced and this is why their hair goes grey.) But all the time the hair cells are producing more and more of the strong hair protein, and by the time the cells get to the surface of the skin, they have been choked off by all the protein building up inside them. By now, they are completely dead, and they bind onto each other in a very striking pattern.

Each hair has quite a soft core, surrounded by thousands of strands of hair protein (the fibres which give the hair its strength). To protect these fibres, more of the protein forms a 'scale' arrangement, a bit like a fir cone. The 'scales' are wrapped tightly around the centre shaft of the hair in a covering called the cuticle, which acts almost like armour plating.

You can actually feel the cuticle in your own hair if you hold one of the longer ones straight out from your head. Lightly moisten the finger and thumb on your other hand and gently grip the hair as near to your head as possible. Then draw the finger and thumb along the hair towards your other hand. It should feel smooth all the way, because you will be sliding over the cuticle scales, smoothing them down the way they are designed to lie naturally, just as if you were closing a fir cone from its base. Now slide your finger and thumb back along the hair towards your head. You should be able to feel the resistance from the cuticle scales as they are made to stand up on end.

Your hair grows because the continuing production of new hair cells below the skin, deep inside the follicle, pushes more and more dead cells and hair protein out of the skin. If that pushing goes on at an

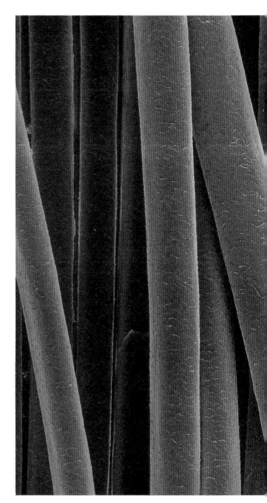

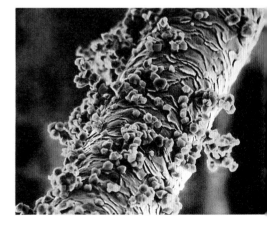

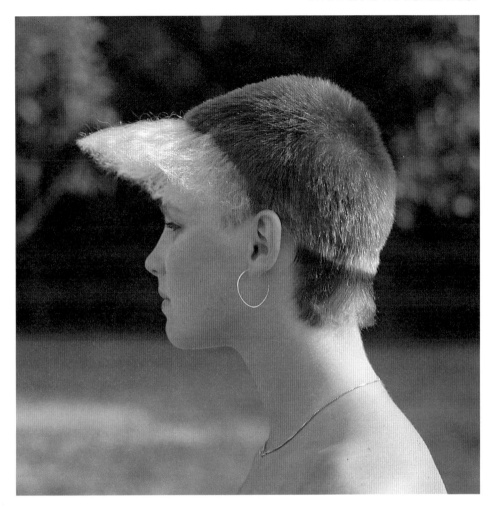

People often tell us more about themselves with their hairstyles than with their clothes. And we can easily jump to the wrong conclusions because of our own prejudices about what a hairstyle implies. Would you think this girl more likely to be a doctor, a lawyer or a secretary?

Compare the clean, strong, natural hairs (above left) with the one being invaded by destructive shampoo molecules (below left).

even rate all around the hair shaft, you get a straight hair. But if you have inherited the kind of hair follicles and cells where the 'push' is uneven, then dead cells and protein build up on one side more than the other, causing the hair to bend and twist – which is how some people come to have a natural curl.

If you cut or shave your hair you only get rid of the dead part above the surface of the skin, so the activity in the hair follicle is not affected at all. This means you cannot stop hair growing or make it grow thicker

11

or bushier by frequent cutting; only old wives' tales will tell you otherwise.

Left to its own devices, your hair will grow 6 inches every year. That may not sound like much, until you think what you would look like at 20 years old if you never had a haircut! But in practice you are very unlikely to find anyone with 10-foot-long hair on their 20th birthday. That is because every single hair on our bodies has a limited lifespan, after which it simply falls out. Then, after the papilla has rested for about 100 days, a new hair begins growing in its place. Not all our hair starts to grow at the same time, so some hairs are always falling out, even when your hair is quite healthy. It also explains why your hairs are all different lengths – they are all at different stages of development. (You can see this easily if you look at the back of your hand or arm.)

Just how long our hairs grow before falling out depends on the pattern we inherit from our parents. Our inherited characteristics also control the stage at which, in some people, certain papillae stop renewing the fallen hairs. This is why some of us go partially or completely bald. And because it is a natural inherited characteristic, there is no simple and safe way to cure this type of baldness. There are some forms of temporary baldness or hair-loss which can be reversed: alopecia, for instance, when whole patches of hair fall out because of stress perhaps; or the heavy hair-losses some women experience during pregnancy. But these conditions are best treated with the help of your doctor, and certainly do not need expensive independently advertised treatments.

In fact it seems that the less you do to your hair, the healthier it will be. Even washing and drying damages the cuticles and can tear at some of the inner fibres of protein. Things get even worse if you bleach and dye your hair. The chemicals destroy the natural substances in the hair which help bind it together, and fill the weakened hair with colouring chemicals, preventing the cuticle scales from closing up properly. Straightening curly hair, or curling straight hair with a perm does even more damage. Tough chemical bonds between the protein fibres have to be broken so that the hair can be set in a new position before the bonds are re-formed. Some of these bonds are never re-formed, making the hair permanently weaker. Once the perm has grown out, re-perming only weakens it further.

Because of all these problems, one brave volunteer agreed to see what would happen if she did nothing to her hair except run lukewarm water through it occasionally – no shampoo, no heavy towelling or blow drying, and no bleach, dye or perms. She found the first 2 weeks easy enough, but by the 4th and 5th week things were pretty intolerable: 'I had to unpeel my hair from my head each morning; and each time I touched my hair I had to wash my hands. My sister said I smelt of sheep!'

But after 6 weeks her natural hair-cleansing chemicals settled down, and after 8 weeks she was convinced that her hair was healthier than it had ever been. The dandruff she used to have completely disappeared, and her scalp felt clean and comfortable. She was so pleased with the condition of her hair that she resolved to 'leave it to nature' in the future – a very positive recommendation for a minimum maintenance thatched roof.

PROGRAMMING THE CONTROL ROOM

Moving from the hair, below the skull we find what must surely be the most vital part of our body – the brain. It is only when the brain stem dies that we clinically certify a person as dead. Without a functioning brain stem, the automatic processes of breathing and blood circulation – and so living itself – cannot take place. And beyond that, we need our brains to help us recognise sensations, learn from them, and decide what to do about them. So it is perhaps surprising that, in one respect at least, our brain is distinctly fallible.

One of the things our brains do is to remember and store information. We know how easy it is to store information electronically; computers and tape-recorders do it all the time on magnetic material. Pass the information through the machine once, and it is there, stored, ready to be recalled whenever we want. The entire works of Shakespeare, all Beethoven's symphonies – they can all be produced at the touch of a button from quite tiny little boxes of electronic circuitry. But our brains are simply not as reliable as that. Although you have passed the previous pages of this book through your brain already, it would be remarkable if you could put the book down and recall everything you have read word for word.

So why have we evolved what seems to be a less than perfect brain?

We need to discover how the control room in our citadel is programmed if we want to find some sort of answer to that question. We certainly do not have the equivalent of yards of empty magnetic tape onto which we just record everything that happens to us. Memory expert Creighton Carvello, for instance, can remember the value of the mathematical constant 'pi' to an incredible 20 000 or more decimal places. It takes him 9 hours and 10 minutes to recite it; but it took him just over 2 years to learn it. If our brains worked like tape-recorders, he could simply have loaded a 10-hour 'tape' and read through the numbers once. Instead, he had to find another way of learning them. Why not try a small memory feat for yourself? Read the 19 letters on the next line slowly and carefully over the next 20 seconds, then shut the book and try to write them down in order:

CMTMYHSIEUOTLASIEOR

Now check to see how well you did. If you got more than the first six or seven right, you did very well. That is about the most that an average person can expect to remember. In a moment you can repeat

13

the test with the same 19 letters in a different order, and this time you will get them all right with no trouble at all. (So as not to give the game away, we have printed the two lists on different pages.) What you are really trying to discover is why you can remember the letters so easily this time. Ready? Then look at the next line and start your watch.

THISISACLUETOMEMORY

Suddenly it is all rather obvious! Once the letters are arranged in a meaningful pattern it is easy to remember all 19 in the right order. Our brains do not simply record random information like a computer; they look for an association between all the things we are trying to remember, and make use of that association in the act of memorising.

If recognising a pattern is so important, you may wonder whether recognising and remembering are all part of the same mental process. Interestingly enough, scientists recently discovered that memory involves activity all over the outer surface of the brain, or cortex. What seems to be happening, all in a fraction of a second, is a whole sequence of events. First, the eye sees the row of letters on the page, the information travels down the optic nerve from the eye, and this stimulates the visual cortex at the back of the brain, to 'register' the sensation from the eye. The 'pattern' of the sensation is then 'reviewed' in the temporal cortex, to see if it can be identified as something we have experienced before. In this case it tells us that they are letters which make up a meaningful set of words. Then the parietal cortex perhaps distinguishes the separate words so that we understand the sentence 'THIS IS A CLUE TO MEMORY' even

though there were no spaces between the words.

Each of these bits of information does not get remembered on its own. Deep inside the brain, in the hippocampus, a kind of encoding goes on – and the result is what we remember. But the whole memorised fact is not stored as a single piece of data; instead each key detail is sent back and stored at the site where it was first experienced – this time in a kind of shorthand note to save space. And the combination of these 'shorthand notes' makes up the complete memory.

You can test this for yourself quite easily. Try to remember what you were doing at exactly this time one week ago. Think aloud as you work it out. Your chain of thought will probably go something like this:

'Was I watching TV then?' . . . 'No, I was still doing my homework.'
'Why was I working late?' . . . 'To finish my English essay.'
'Which essay did I have to finish?' . . . 'The one on Romeo and Juliet.'

Only after all these thoughts will you say 'This time last week I was writing an essay on Romeo and Juliet', because you have to 'explore' the memorised shorthand notes in each section of the cortex before you can piece the whole thing together again.

The great advantage of this kind of memory system is that you can grope your way towards information without even knowing where it is stored. Having got this far down the line with the subject of the essay, you may be able to explore further lines of enquiry to remember the main points in the essay and perhaps some of the quotations you used to support them.

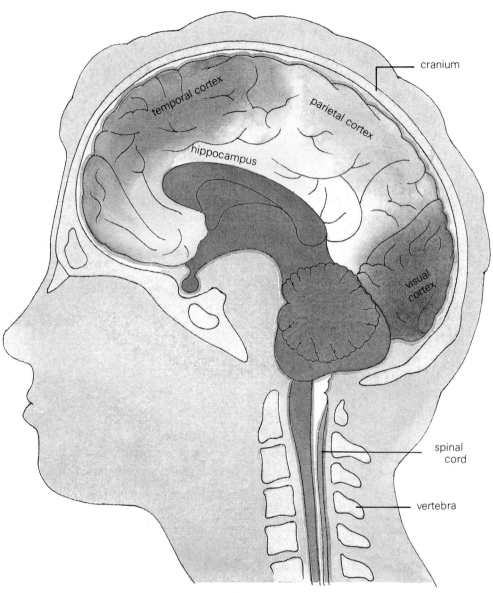

cranium

temporal cortex

parietal cortex

hippocampus

visual cortex

spinal cord

vertebra

But if, like a computer, you simply stored your memory of what you were doing last week in one file, details of your homework in another, and quotations from *Romeo and Juliet* in a third, you could only get at the information if you remembered the name of each file and where it was kept. Very quick and efficient if you happen to

SIMPLIFIED DIAGRAM SHOWING MAIN AREAS OF THE BRAIN

15

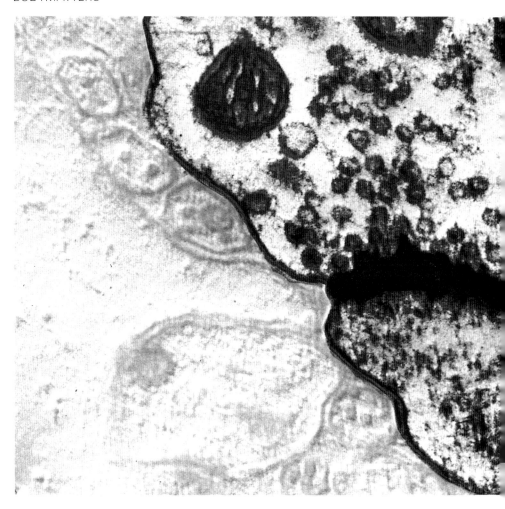

remember, but totally useless if you forget. Short of running through your entire life's memories until you find what you want, the information would be irretrievably lost. The slightly slower, more imperfect memory system has the enormous advantage that we can usually find things soon enough, without having to know a file name or a code word. We simply follow the pathways in our brain that connect various experiences together.

Another way of seeing this exploration system in action is to reflect on how we learn the words of a part in a play. We repeat them to ourselves over and over again. At first we can only remember bits here and there, not the whole thing. With several repetitions we get better, until eventually we remember all the words in the play. It is as if we are trying to locate the appropriate parts of the cortex to store each bit of this complex memory, and then cutting a pathway to join them all together. Each time we make the journey, the pathway gets a little clearer, and so progress gets easier. This theory is con-

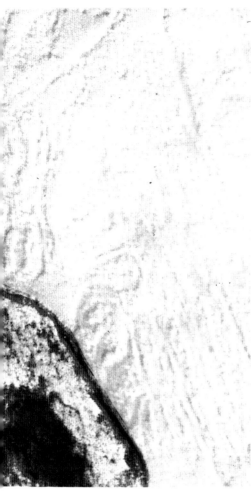

This is a synapse, or junction, between two nerve cells, magnified 17 600 times. The red band is where all the chemical exchanges are taking place while a message is transferred from one cell to the other.

meaningful words, or the events of a week ago into ways of retrieving specific information about homework and *Romeo and Juliet*. We are also capable of associating an image with quite an unlikely second image. Imagine a tree with legs running down the road. Not too hard, is it? But you have never seen one, so how did you think of it? A computer could not have associated two disconnected pieces of information in that way, but we can. That is the genius of the human brain; we can think and imagine creatively. It may be a long way from a tree with legs to the works of Shakespeare or a Beethoven symphony, but being able to think creatively is the most vital ingredient in any artist's original work. It is only when that creative association of ideas has taken place in a human brain that it can be reproduced on paper. It can of course then be copied and fed into a computer's memory; but it could never have originated there.

But even if you will never be a Van Gogh, creative association of ideas is also very helpful in improving your day-to-day memory. Suppose you want to remember a list of 10 objects: MELON, BUTTERFLY, RIVER, HELICOPTER, ENVELOPE, RIBBON, PETTICOAT, PENCIL, CAMEL and LORRY. Close the book now and have a go at recalling them in order . . .

. . . Not much success? Well, try making a crazy pictorial association between the objects. If you find it hard to conjure up pictures in your mind, just turn the page – where you'll find we've done it all for you.

firmed by scientific studies of the synapses (or junctions between nerves) during a particular act of memorising. At first the chemical activity is vigorous and chaotic, but as the memorising goes on, the activity dies down as if the pathway is now well trodden and needs no more clearing.

But we do not have to make and follow well-trodden pathways all the time. Another bonus of the exploration way of remembering things is our fertile imagination. We do not just associate the letters THISISACLUETOMEMORY into

17

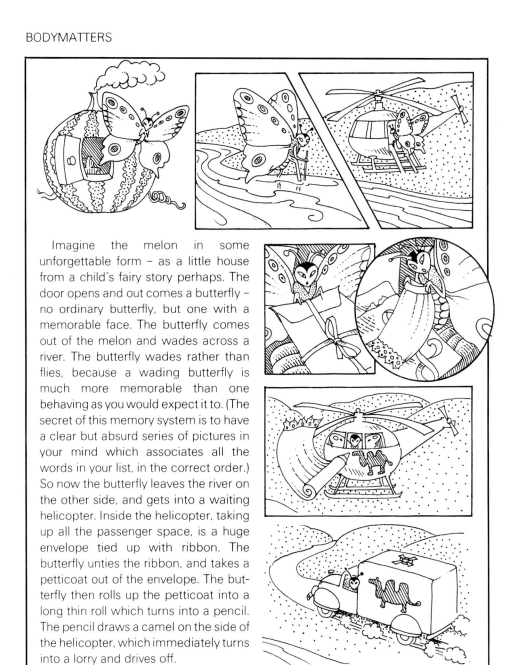

Imagine the melon in some unforgettable form – as a little house from a child's fairy story perhaps. The door opens and out comes a butterfly – no ordinary butterfly, but one with a memorable face. The butterfly comes out of the melon and wades across a river. The butterfly wades rather than flies, because a wading butterfly is much more memorable than one behaving as you would expect it to. (The secret of this memory system is to have a clear but absurd series of pictures in your mind which associates all the words in your list, in the correct order.) So now the butterfly leaves the river on the other side, and gets into a waiting helicopter. Inside the helicopter, taking up all the passenger space, is a huge envelope tied up with ribbon. The butterfly unties the ribbon, and takes a petticoat out of the envelope. The butterfly then rolls up the petticoat into a long thin roll which turns into a pencil. The pencil draws a camel on the side of the helicopter, which immediately turns into a lorry and drives off.

If you now close the book and recall the series of pictures in your mind, you should have no trouble remembering all 10 words in the correct order. Just why visual images are so useful to us when we associate ideas is not quite so easy to explain; but it is undoubtedly a very useful technique for programming our memory.

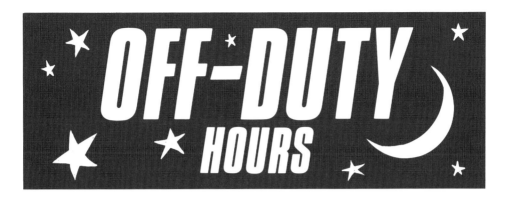

OFF-DUTY HOURS

C onsidering that we spend about a third of our lives asleep, it is remarkable how little scientists actually know about why our bodies need to be unconscious and off-duty in this way. They have managed to find out quite a lot about our surprisingly varied and busy sleep patterns, and what makes us fall asleep and wake up, but they are no nearer to any positive proof of what sleep does for us in the first place.

To study sleep, scientists can wire up

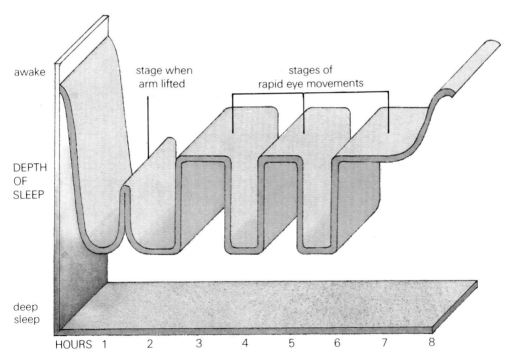

awake

stage when
arm lifted

stages of
rapid eye movements

DEPTH
OF
SLEEP

deep
sleep

HOURS 1   2   3   4   5   6   7   8

This simple graph records the pattern of a volunteer's sleep from the moment they first fell asleep to the time they woke up 8 hours later. It is reasonably typical of how any of us might spend a good night's sleep.

the brain of a volunteer before he or she drops off, and monitor the brain's electrical activity all through sleep. They can also observe any bodily changes, such as distinctive movements, muscle tone, changes in breathing pattern and so on. By seeing which brain activity changes coincide with which physical activity, they can put together quite a detailed picture of a typical sleep pattern.

When you first start to fall asleep the amount of electrical activity in the brain decreases, but it never stops altogether. You obviously need some activity to ensure that you keep breathing, for example, even though you are unconscious and asleep. You also need some form of sensory awareness in order to respond to danger or disturbance and wake up. Essentially these central life-supporting activities follow a smooth regular pattern. Your brain activity therefore slows down from the fast, chaotic, scurrying collection of electrical signals typical of a fully alert condition to a slower, more orderly and rhythmical set of readings. An experienced technician will be able to recognise these patterns on the volunteer's printout, and see when he or she changes from one pattern to the other, or maybe hovers in between. Most volunteers will cover the complete range, or in other words fall into a deep sleep, within half an hour of nodding off.

One of the physical effects of this deep sleep is that our muscles become completely limp. The graph shows when this was confirmed with our volunteer, by lifting one arm and gently letting it drop, once he or she had been in deep sleep for about half an hour. It also confirmed that there was nothing wrong with the sensory alertness of the sleeping brain; the activity increased as soon as the arm was lifted,

and the sleep became much shallower, even though the volunteer did not wake up and rapidly went back into deep sleep.

After 2½ hours, the volunteer went into a light, shallower kind of sleep quite naturally, and this time stayed there for about an hour. And something very noticeable happened during that period. Suddenly the volunteer's eyeballs started rolling around under the eyelids. This happens to all of us, and is known as Rapid Eye Movement sleep, or REM sleep. If you wake someone up during REM sleep, they will always say that they were dreaming at the time. Not everyone remembers their dreams when they finally wake up naturally; and this explains why some people swear they never dream. But sleep testing in the laboratory confirms that every single one of us does.

In fact we go into REM sleep several times each night during our periods of light sleep, so we do quite a lot of dreaming. And also, as the graph shows, the periods of deep sleep tend to become shorter and the periods of shallow sleep tend to become longer, as the night progresses. One possible reason for this pattern is that we need to relax the whole body during deep sleep so that our muscles and brain can be refreshed, ready for another day's activity. This is the most urgent role of sleep so we go into deep sleep first, in case we are woken early. All we then miss in the shallower sleep, the theory goes, is the chance to sift, filter and store the data lodged in our brains during the period before we fell asleep. Dreaming could be a part of this essential information organisation – we often remember dreaming of events from the previous day in strange illogical arrangements, as if we are trying to discover associations between them. And

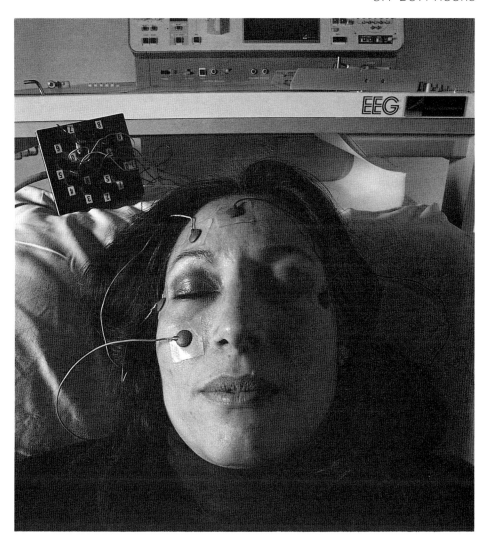

many people wake up with a solution to a problem clearly in their minds, when it had eluded them the evening before. So one explanation of our sleep pattern might be that shallower sleep is used to prepare the memory and computing side of the brain only, while deep sleep gets the brain and body ready for action and energy-demanding work.

But if sleep is so obviously beneficial, how and why do we sometimes manage

A sleep volunteer under observation, wired up to sensitive machinery which will record every change in muscle tone, brain activity, etc.

to do without it? We clearly do not like to miss our sleep, since we feel really tired and grotty without it, but it would be hopeless if we fell asleep automatically at some pre-set time. You could, for instance, be delayed getting home one night and find

21

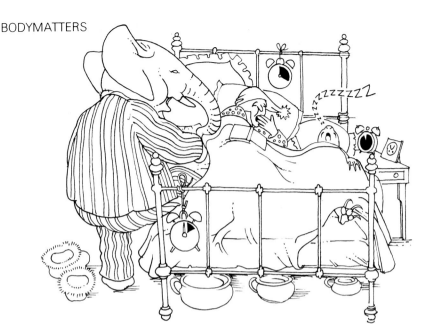

yourself driving down a motorway at your usual bedtime, when falling asleep would be disastrous!

What appears to switch sleep on and off is the balance between the sleep-inducing and alertness chemicals which are produced naturally in our bodies. We normally sleep at night and stay awake during the day because daylight seems to trigger the pineal gland in the brain to produce alertness hormones, and this is why we tend to sleep least in the summer when the days are longest. If we are deprived of sleep, then the brain gets flooded with sleep-inducing hormones to cancel out the effect of the alertness hormones (produced by the daylight), and we can sleep during the day to catch up. But if we need to stay awake, despite being short of sleep, we can in turn overcome the sleep-inducing hormones by producing other alertness hormones like adrenalin. The supply of these alertness hormones is triggered off by danger as well as our own determination to concentrate and stay alert, and this explains how

An elephant would wake up at least 2 hours before you, and 15 hours before a sloth!

we can manage quite difficult tasks even when we are desperately tired. In this situation, we produce enough short-lived alertness hormones to hold back the effects of the sleep-inducing hormones which are building up in the brain. But once the immediate challenge is over, and our lives settle into a more routine, comfortable, safe pattern the sleep chemicals dominate and we begin to nod off.

Despite all this knowledge of how our sleep system works, much of it still remains a complete mystery. If people force themselves to manage on 6 hours' sleep a night, some of them find that they actually feel better for it. And a few people seem to thrive on only 2 or 3 hours a night. Elephants seem to want 4 hours a night, yet the three-toed sloth appears to need at least 19 hours in every 24. Perhaps you should sleep on these puzzling facts if you want to discover some explanations . . .

KEEPING ON THE LOOKOUT

There is no doubt that the most alert sentries in the citadel are our eyes. They are constantly scanning everything before us, sending a never-ending stream of information to our central control room, the brain. And while touch, taste, smell and hearing can be just as involved in monitoring our surroundings, it

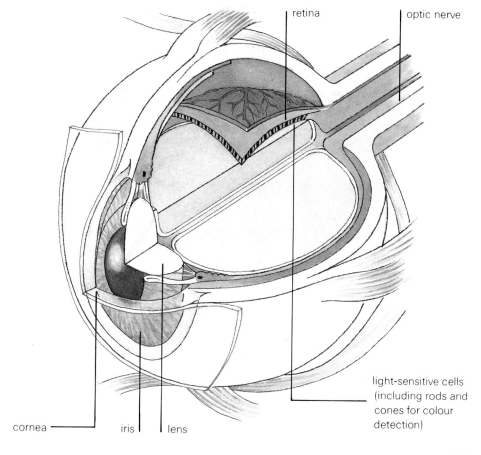

retina

optic nerve

light-sensitive cells (including rods and cones for colour detection)

cornea

iris

lens

is usually sight which gives us our all-important first impressions. If our eyes are deceived, then, more often than not, so are we.

In fact it is amazingly easy for our eyes to be deceived. Just take a look at this set of squares:

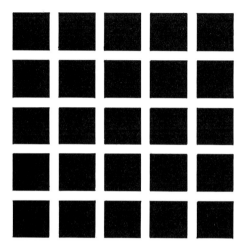

If you stare at the page hard, you cannot fail to 'see' the grey dots at the corners of the black squares, filling the white 'cross-roads'. But they are not really there, printed on the page. It is all an optical illusion.

The reason our eyes can be fooled in this and many other ways is because of the way they receive images of things. Whereas a camera records visual information chemically on film, the eye turns it into electrical signals, so that it can be sent along the optic nerve to the brain for processing. We may react immediately, decide to store the information and do something about it later or perhaps ignore it altogether. Whatever we do, it is in the making and retaining of the electrical signals while we look at the squares that the deception occurs. To understand it, we need to follow the workings of the eye

from the beginning.

Light is reflected from the page of the book, and specifically the squares pattern, into the pupil – the 'black hole' in the eye. The pupil changes size according to the amount of light available. In poor light it widens to let in enough light for us to see clearly; in bright light it narrows, so that we are not dazzled.

The pupil does this in exactly the same way, and for exactly the same reason, as a camera with an adjustable aperture. By allowing only the ideal amount of light into the camera, we ensure that a properly exposed photograph is taken. The iris in the eye – the distinctively coloured part – ensures that the right amount of visual information goes to the back of the eye. Both the camera and the eye, however, have to adjust the image before it is registered, either on the photographic film or on the back of the eye. Otherwise we would see only a blurred outline.

Once the right amount of light has entered the eye or camera, it has to be focused to produce a clear image. But while the focusing part of the camera lens is made up of separate solid pieces of glass, the lens in the eye is a single soft, transparent, fluid-filled sac. Focusing the camera lens means varying the distance between the glass elements, whereas focusing the eye involves muscles stretching or 'fattening' the elastic sac. The nearer things are to your eyes, the fatter the lens has to be to get them into focus. And the whole process of focusing turns the image upside down – you can see what happens with a magnifying glass as a lens.

The upside-down focused image falls onto a kind of screen, the retina, at the back of the eye. It is paper-thin, and contains various kinds of light-sensitive cells.

These cells respond to the image by sending electrical impulses to the optic nerve, which carries the information to the brain. Some of these light-sensitive cells are good at sensing colour, and some of them specialise in distinguishing light from dark. When we look at the black squares, the information from the cells detecting the darkness of the black squares gets confused with information from the cells registering the white spaces between them. And this is why we 'see' the grey spots.

Because the eye is such a delicate precision instrument, it has to be carefully protected and regularly cleaned. The outside of the eyeball is a transparent layer of skin, which is kept clean and healthy by repeated wash and brush-up routines as we blink – allowing our eyelashes and the cleansing fluid produced by the tear ducts to do their work. When serious irritants affect the eye – like the vapour from chopped onions – a full-scale weep is needed to wash away the sulphuric acid produced in the watery film on the eyeball. And emotions can affect our eyes too. No prizes for knowing that we cry for emotional reasons, but did you know that the pupil varies in size, partly in response to how much we like what we are looking at? When two lovers meet, their pupils get bigger as they look into each other's eyes.

The most common problems with our eyes involve the focusing system. If the back of the eye is too near the lens, then you will be long-sighted. And if the back of the eye is too far away from the lens then you will be short-sighted. Fortunately, of course, both these problems are easily solved with contact lenses or glasses. And even people with perfect sight in their youth are likely to need glasses as they grow older. Because the lens sac becomes less elastic with age, we find it harder to focus quickly, finely, and with the same wide range.

It is remarkable what can be done for rarer and more dangerous eye disorders. For instance, if a cataract makes the clear fluid inside the lens become more and more cloudy, the whole lens can be removed by surgery, and glasses used to restore limited focusing abilities. If the retina at the back of the eye gets detached or damaged, it can be examined with light shone into the eye and surgery performed with a laser beam so that the rest of the eye does not have to be cut or damaged in any way. Diabetics are particularly vulnerable to retina damage because their retinas can become very crowded with tiny thin blood vessels. If these extra-fragile blood vessels burst, they could bleed into the eyeball, causing sudden blindness. So diabetics should have their eyes checked regularly; and if need be, the vulnerable blood vessels can be destroyed by laser treatment.

There is one other possible defect you might want to check for yourself. Look at the circles full of coloured dots on the next page. All female readers and 92 per cent of the males will see the numbers 5, 6, 7 and 8 easily enough; but 8 per cent of men inherit colour blindness, and they will not be able to see some or all of them.

You cannot correct colour blindness, but it is really no great handicap if you do turn out to be colour-blind. It simply means that the rods and cones (the light-sensitive cells in the retina which detect the primary colours, red, green and blue) are incorrectly balanced, or maybe one set is not working properly. This makes it impossible to distinguish between some colours.

White light is made up equally of all

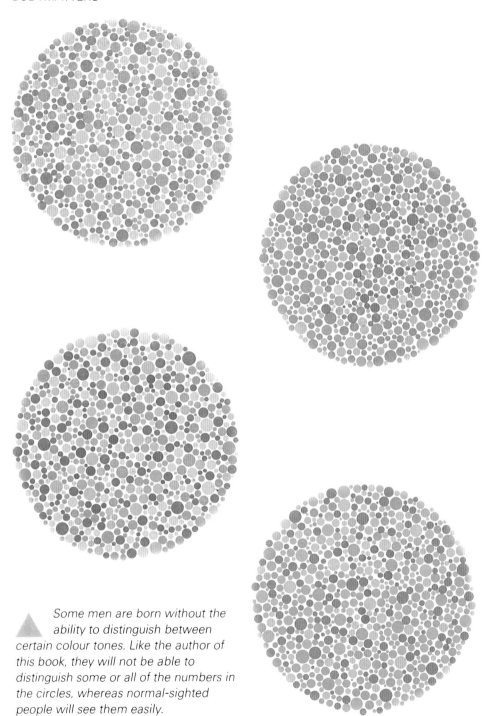

Some men are born without the ability to distinguish between certain colour tones. Like the author of this book, they will not be able to distinguish some or all of the numbers in the circles, whereas normal-sighted people will see them easily.

three primary colours, and if the cones and rods in the retina are equally saturated with light, a message is encoded and sent to the brain so that we see white. We see other colours when the cones are not equally saturated by the light; but if only the red ones are saturated, we see red. If there is some saturation of all three we would probably see some shade of brown, depending on the degree to which each is saturated. With all the range of combinations available, we are able to see the whole spectrum of possible colours the world can offer us.

Just to show you that it all boils down to the saturation of rods and cones, try this little test. Stare hard at the green elephant below for at least 30 seconds, concentrating on the spot on the elephant's tummy. Then look away immediately at a clean sheet of white paper.

Now what are you seeing? A pink elephant, of course! The reason is that if you stare at anything long enough, you will keep an image of it on the retina for a short while after you finish looking at it – this is called 'visual persistence'. And if you see something which is in one of the primary colours – in this case green – then the rods and cones which respond to that colour get fully saturated, and eventually switch off temporarily. So the image you see, thanks to visual persistence, is given a colour by the other rods and cones (in this case the red and blue ones), which is why you see a purply-pink elephant!

Which all goes to prove, not that pink elephants are real, but that our usually highly reliable eyes can deceive us. And that's why it's useful to have other sensory systems to check whatever our eyes tell us as they keep a lookout.

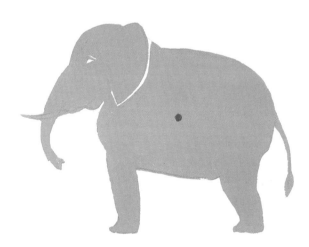

OUR COMMUNICATIONS NETWORK

O ur eyes, and every other organ in the sensory system, can only serve us properly if what they sense can be relayed to the brain. The brain either stores the information in our memory, or rejects it as unimportant; it also decides whether or not immediate action is required. If we need to go into action, then messages have to be sent to the appropriate tissues – bone, blood, muscles and so on. These messages are sent from the sense organs to the brain, and from the brain to the tissues, along the appropriate nerves.

The nervous system in our bodies is rather like the electrical wiring in buildings. Like wiring, the nerves take electrical signals from the control room to every corner of the citadel and back again. But nerves do not conduct a current from one point to the next along a single strand of metal, though we often say that a cool,

courageous person has 'nerves of steel'.

To understand how our nerves actually work, it might be more helpful to think of Guy Fawkes and gunpowder, rather than modern electrical wiring. The way messages travel from one nerve cell to the next is rather like a flame travelling along a trail of gunpowder. The end of the trail is lit, and the flame leaps from one clump of powder to the next, until it reaches the powder keg at the end. In the same way,

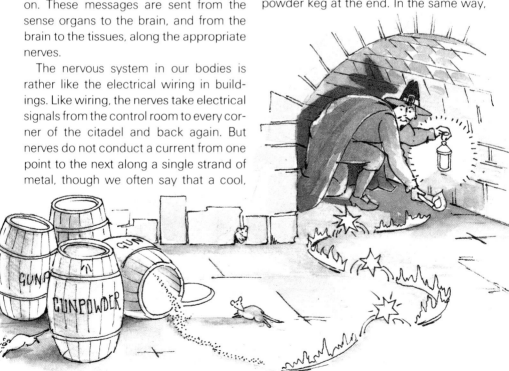

messages jump from one nerve cell to the next before reaching their destination.

Nerve cells, or neurones, may be microscopically thin but they can also be extraordinarily long. There is one, for instance, as long as your leg – stretching from the big toe to the base of the spinal cord. There it connects with another nerve cell, which in turn is connected to another, and so on, until a chain from the big toe to the brain is completed. In the same way, chains of nerve cells run from the brain to all the other parts of the body and back; what we would call a nerve is usually a bundle of these chains. The complete network is arranged so that almost all of them pass through the hollow part of the back-

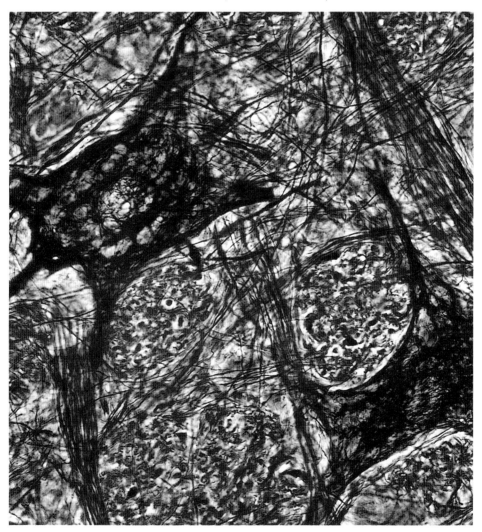

These two neurones, magnified about 200 times, are amongst the hundred thousand million found in a mature healthy brain.

bone as part of the spinal cord. Only the nerves in the head connect directly to the brain without passing through the spinal cord.

Like all living cells, each of the nerve cells in these chains contains a nucleus inside a cell body. But in neurones this cell body is extended into a long, thin, fibre-like shape called the axon. It is the axon which stretches between one nerve cell and the next, and it is surrounded by a protective sheath – a kind of white, fatty covering called myelin. This covering is not totally watertight but it still keeps the axon bathed in fluid. At intervals along the length of the axon, the myelin narrows, and there is a sort of gateway between one bit of the axon and the next. It is at these points that the message being transmitted along a nerve fibre has to 'leap across' to the next bit of axon just as a flame 'leaps' from one bit of gunpowder to the next.

It is all to do with the electrical properties of chemicals. The axon is continually pumping sodium out into the fluid between itself and the myelin, leaving the inside of the axon fairly rich in potassium. When a message (encoded as electrical

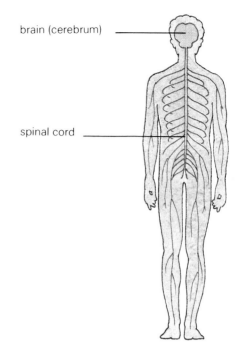

brain (cerebrum)

spinal cord

SIMPLIFIED PLAN OF NERVOUS SYSTEM

 A: Imagine stubbing your right big toe.
B: Chemicals called kinins are released, setting off a message to the brain from the toe which we recognise as pain; this in turn means messages are sent to other parts of the body. For instance, our face grimaces and our right hand grabs the toe – all before we are really conscious of doing anything.
C: Then we begin to send messages we are conscious of: to position our body as comfortably as possible while we rub the toe better, for instance.

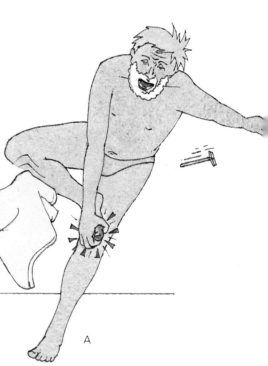

A

30

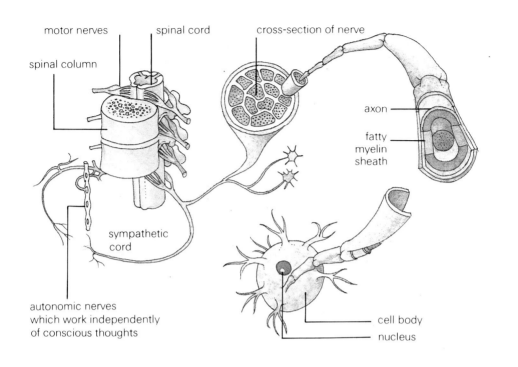

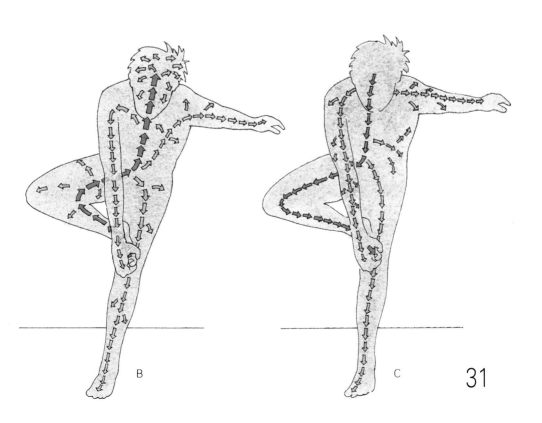

31

impulses) reaches the first bit of the axon, the electrical balance between the two chemicals is changed. The sodium and potassium therefore start to change places in order to adjust it, and this opens the gateway to the next bit of the axon. The impulse then moves into the new section of axon, where the next gateway is opened in the same way. Eventually, when the impulse reaches the end of the nerve cell, it is transferred to the next nerve cell in similar fashion, and so on. Finally it reaches the brain, which is itself a whole complex of neurones especially arranged to handle the reading, storing and answering of messages, rather like a highly sophisticated cross between a telephone exchange and a computer.

You can measure the speed at which an impulse travels along a nerve fibre – around 150 miles per hour is pretty typical and healthy. It never travels as fast as electricity, even though the speed does vary in different people and different parts of the body. The less leaky the myelin sheath and the bigger the diameter of the axon, the faster the impulse will travel. But 150 miles per hour is quite fast enough for our purposes. After all, the brain needs to get a clear message it can decode and think about, and it then has to send out a reply. We would not want to overburden the poor thing; it only contains 100 000 000 000 neurones of its own when fully mature at the age of 18. And from then on, they die off faster than we can replace them; on balance we lose about 1000 a day for the rest of our lives!

HEARING THINGS
AND STAYING STEADY

Our ears act as very good supporting sentries to our eyes when it comes to guarding our citadel. They can alert us to look in a particular direction or confirm that our eyes really have seen, say, a rattlesnake, by hearing a hiss or a sinister rattle. What is less immediately obvious is the way our ears help us know where we stand. Rather like spirit levels, they can immediately detect when we are standing at an angle or about to topple off a wobbling bicycle. And strangely enough, the key to these seemingly unrelated abilities is remarkably similar. They both involve the tiniest of hairs, deep inside the ear.

But before we go exploring those innermost secrets, it is surprising to discover just how useful even the outer, weirdly shaped, flappy bits are. Believe it or not, every peculiar twist and turn of their shape helps us not only to funnel sounds into our ears, but also to identify the precise place from which the sound is coming. We'll begin our journey into the ear by travelling alongside a sound as it finds its way in.

First we need to know exactly what a sound is. Try holding a page of a newspaper loosely at the bottom corners, and letting the top fall gently against your slightly opened lips. If you speak or make a sound without moving your lips, you can feel the paper vibrating against your mouth. In other words, sounds are disturbances in the air around us; and whenever anything makes a noise, it sets up vibrations or sound waves which travel away from it in all directions.

If we are in hearing distance of the sound, those vibrations will eventually reach our ears. And just as the newspaper's vibrations were gently detected by our lips, so the sound's vibrations will be even more subtly noticed by the outer fleshy part of our ear. They will not have a clue as to what the sound means; all they have to do is tell us it is there. And depending on how it strikes whichever parts of the hills and valleys, ridges and slopes of that outer ear trumpet, messages will go back to the brain to say the sound is, broadly speaking, to the front or back of us, to the left or right, above or below our ears, or straight in between them. We can only pinpoint the location of the sound with any real accuracy later on, when it is analysed in detail inside the inner ear. The brain locates a sound by comparing messages from both ears – so if you are deaf in one ear you will have a poor idea of where sounds are coming from – but the first clues still come from the peculiarly shaped funnel which guides the sound into our ear canals.

33

These ear canals are the hollow tubes that collect wax, and which you can try to pick and poke with your fingers. Fortunately fingers have been specially designed so that they do not quite fit! Otherwise you could end up doing damage to the delicately stretched thin piece of skin which covers the inner end of the canal, the eardrum. If you were daft enough to try, you could reach the eardrum by poking something thinner than a finger into the ear canal. But you would be extremely stupid, because it is all too easy to damage the eardrum, causing chronic pain at the least and possibly irreversible damage and deafness at the worst.

The eardrum has to be very delicate because it detects the vibrations of a sound exactly as the newspaper did. By vibrating itself, it passes on the pattern of the sound wave to a chain of three bones inside the middle ear. (These tiny bones are linked to the cochlea, or inner ear.) The eardrum and the chain of bones are vibrated, and slightly amplify the vibrations before passing them on to the inner ear.

Unlike the rest of the ear, the inner ear does not contain any air. From here on in, the vibrations of sounds are carried through the fluids which fill the long inner passage of the spiral-shaped cochlea. The

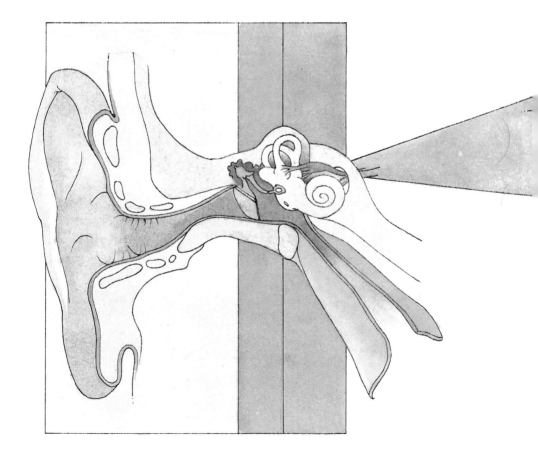

whole cochlea is tiny but all along the coiled passage there are thousands and thousands of tiny hairs. Rather like the strings in a piano (which vibrate according to which notes you play), the hairs in the cochlea all respond to different speeds or frequencies of sound. This means that a complex set of sounds, like a snake hiss and rattle, or a human voice singing or speaking a series of words, will enter the ear as a series of sound waves over a period of time. As each sound wave is experienced, certain hair cells in the cochlea are vibrated. This in turn sends a sequence of electrical impulses along the auditory nerves to the brain, where the precise nature of the sounds can be recognised and interpreted.

The louder the sound, the more the delicate hair cells in the cochlea are shaken and vibrated. They can be shaken so hard that they weaken and collapse, unable to respond any more to loud sounds. This is a kind of deafness which we can all avoid, by not subjecting our ears to continuous, relentless loud noise. All you heavy metal music fans, please note! In fact prolonged exposure to any loud noise is dangerous, which is why you should wear ear defenders when working in noisy surroundings.

Deafness will also occur if the system breaks down at an earlier point – if the eardrum is broken, or the chain of three bones is damaged, for instance. But even then, you can retain some degree of hearing as long as vibrations can somehow reach the cochlea – if part of the drum still vibrates, for example, or the bone chain functions in a limited way, or the bone of the skull next to the ear vibrates sufficiently for the cochlea to pick up the vibrations. In these cases a hearing aid can amplify sounds to the point where the vibrations are more easily detected. But if the cochlea is not working, then a hearing aid cannot help. The only other possibility, which does not work for everyone, is to implant an artificial cochlea. This is an incredibly clever electronic device which can be programmed from a computer outside the body, but it falls far short of the real cochlea in its range and sophistication.

If we go behind the cochlea we find, attached to it, the one part of the ear we have yet to explore – the semicircular canals. These are filled with fluid and hairs, just like the cochlea, but they have nothing to do with hearing. The three semicircular canals are set at right angles

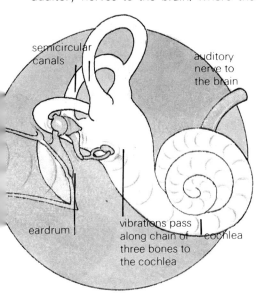

semicircular canals

auditory nerve to the brain

eardrum

vibrations pass along chain of three bones to the cochlea

cochlea

▲ *The middle ear contains the chain of three bones – called the malleus, incus and stapes – which link the eardrum to the cochlea. Together with the three semicircular canals, the cochlea makes up the inner ear.*

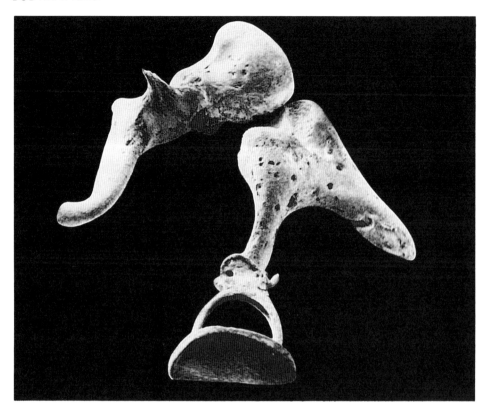

▲ *The malleus (hammer) bone 'strikes' the incus (anvil) bone, which vibrates the stapes (stirrup).*

to each other, and help us keep our balance. Whatever position we adopt, whether lying down or standing up, with our heads at whatever angle, at least one of the canals will always be more or less vertical, one more or less horizontal, and the third at right angles to the other two. At any given moment, one canal might detect roughly how far we are leaning forwards or backwards, while the other is more concerned with how far we are leaning to the left or the right. The relative position of the third canal gives us the final information we need to be sure of the precise position of our body, or rather head. And as that changes, so does the relative position of the canals.

As we move, the fluid in the canals is moved around, and this in turn moves little plates of a jelly-like substance at the end of sets of hairs. The movements of these tiny hairs send messages to the brain. These messages vary according to the degree to which the hairs are bent over in the moving fluid, and the brain can interpret them to work out whether we are safely upright, or being spun round and round, or whatever. You can easily tell that the system works: stand on one leg and close your eyes, and try to figure out why, difficult though it may be, you do not fall over! The only possible conclusion is that something other than your eyes must be telling your brain when to correct your

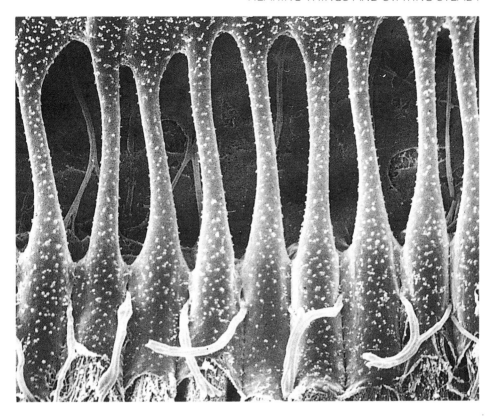

These are some of the tiny hairs inside the cochlea which only vibrate at specific frequencies.

position to ensure that you stay upright.

There are also sacs at the end of the canals which detect the pressure of canal fluid on one or other part of the sac; and this pressure tells us how fast we are moving and in which direction. Try twirling round as fast as you can until you feel giddy! We get this sensation because the brain is receiving conflicting messages – the eyes say we have stopped spinning, while the fluid in the sacs and the semicircular canals is still sloshing around from all the earlier violent movement, keeping the hairs bent over as if we are still in motion. It is a similar confusion of messages from eye and ear which can cause sea, air or car sickness in some people. And this is why some drugs to counter these annoying conditions are designed to 'dampen down' one or both of the conflicting messages to the brain.

When our ears are constantly supplying so much vital information about our position and movement as well as the sounds going on all around us, it is no wonder that even the mildest infection can cause the misery we experience with earache. The strain of trying to ignore the pain of the infection and concentrate on the other information coming from our ears can be extremely tiring. So think twice before you scratch that itch in your ear with a dirty pencil – you could be making things much worse for yourself.

37

SOPHISTICATED AIR CONDITIONING

For many of us, the nose is our single most significant feature when it comes to deciding how attractive we look. Think of how many film stars and pop singers have 'nose jobs'! Interestingly enough, it is not a totally misguided fantasy to think that your nose will affect your love-life; the nose plays a vital part when boy meets girl, but perhaps not in the way you would imagine. When you find someone sexually attractive, believe it or not, your nose swells. This is why couples on honeymoon quite often come home with colds; but more of that later. The main function of the nose is to let us smell things and to prepare the air we breathe for its journey into our lungs. It both cleans and warms the air, so that the delicate lining of the lungs will not be damaged. And the

way the nose goes about this important air-conditioning role is really quite clever.

If you feel your nose, you will find that you can waggle it about quite easily. That is because most of the stiff bit down the middle is not a bone, but a piece of flexible cartilage. It allows the nose to take a few knocks – as it inevitably must, since it sticks right out in front of you – without breaking. And it also separates the two identical halves of the nose, each with its nostril as the ever-open way for air to get in.

Most people imagine that the nose merely contains a couple of funnels leading to the back of the mouth, but the two outer parts are quite cunningly arranged. The hairs you can see massing around the entrance to the nose filter the air as soon

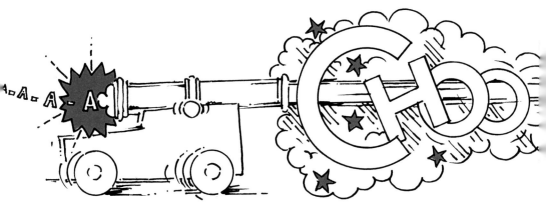

as it gets through the nostril, stopping any solid impurities going any further. Then the air is drawn upwards over the turbinate – a rather bony fold in the nose wall covered in mucous membrane. This membrane is rich in very tiny blood vessels, with delicate thin walls. They are vulnerable to the slightest increase in pressure, which is why nose bleeds occur so easily. But they have to be thin so that the warmth of the blood running through them can be transferred to the incoming air and heat it up. The mucous membrane also supplies mucus to moisten the air. Our lungs like air to be humidified as well as warm!

Most of the time, the air is filtered and warmed and goes on its way without us being conscious of it. But if the turbinate needs to, it can react in two different ways to get rid of unwanted invaders which try to get in along with the air we breathe. First, it can trigger a sneeze. When it is irritated, the membrane quickly sends a message through part of the nervous system over which we have little control, saying that some dirty or infected air is on its way to the lungs and we must get rid of it fast. The muscles of the chest then contract violently, forcing all the air out of the lungs and back up to the mouth and nose.

Because the nostrils are so small, the expelled air is driven through them at enormous speed. This has been measured, and the world record for a sneeze stands at a staggering 103 miles per hour!

The second thing the membrane can do is to bring more blood into the area, since it contains white cells especially designed to fight germs and viruses. These cells are sent out into the nose to do battle in an increased flow of mucus. And because of all the extra blood swelling the membrane, the passage along the turbinate gets narrowed and the nose can redden – hence the all too familiar runny, red, blocked-up nose we get with colds and 'flu. If the nose swells up repeatedly for other reasons, such as when you are spending a lot of time with someone you fancy, the mucous membrane receives a constant rush of blood to engorge it. The theory is that this makes an enticing resting place for cold germs, and so we get all those honeymoon colds.

One thing we notice as soon as our noses are swollen and runny is that we lose our sense of smell. That is because the smelling part of the nose is high up inside the nose and gets blocked off by the extra mucus and swelling. Even with a clear nose, we tend to sniff in delicate

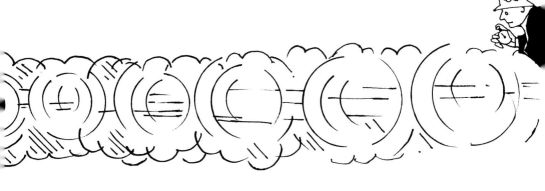

39

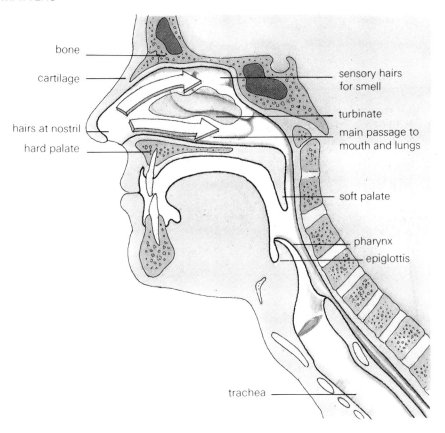

bone
cartilage
hairs at nostril
hard palate

sensory hairs
for smell
turbinate
main passage to
mouth and lungs
soft palate
pharynx
epiglottis
trachea

Normal breathing sends air down the main passage to the lungs; sniffing takes air up past the sensory hairs so that smells can be detected.

The world's most powerful sneezers have actually been timed to discover the fastest sneeze on earth.

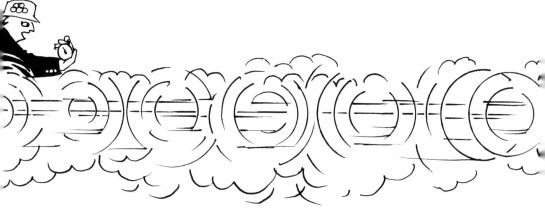

smells deeply if we want to detect what they are. The air carrying the odour has to go up the nostril, past the turbinate, and into another passage (rather like the turbinate) which lies just above it. This passage is lined with rows and rows of small delicate hairs; and each one of them has a special receptor, rather like a lock which can only receive one key. Any smell that enters the nose carries the equivalent of a bunch of keys which are unique to that smell; and each of these keys finds the hair which has the right lock for it. The hairs then send messages to the brain. And the combined information from all of them is a kind of code which the brain quickly unscrambles so that we can recognise the smell.

We use our sense of smell as a vital part of our tasting ability. Get someone to pour you a glass of wine while you are blindfolded with a peg on your nose; then sip the wine and see how difficult it is to recognise it. When you remove the peg you'll realise what a difference your sense of smell makes. But despite its importance, our sense of smell is not nearly as well developed as that of, say, an alsatian. In their much longer noses, they have a hundred times as many of those hairs and receptors as we do – which is why they can be trained as sniffer dogs.

And one last thought on the way our noses affect our personal lives. As well as spoiling honeymoons, they have been accused of being one of the major causes of marital breakdowns and divorce. They are, after all, the organ through which we snore. As we sleep, the muscles in the soft palate area of the mouth and the turbinates in the nose naturally relax. The soft palate and turbinates can then vibrate as you breathe, setting up sound waves which are all too easily amplified in the trumpet shape of the nostrils. Snoring which keeps a partner awake has proved fatal to many a marriage, and there is no simple cure for it. The bigger the nose, the louder the snore tends to be – perhaps one good reason why we humans should not be envious of the long sensitive nose of the alsatian after all!

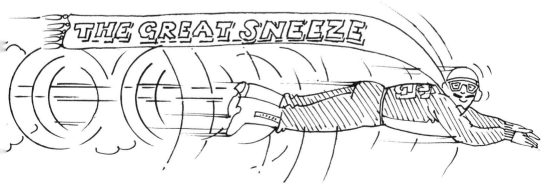

THE TOUGHEST LITTLE TOOLKIT AVAILABLE

There are some really remarkable tests to prove just how tough our teeth are. For instance, if you can cement a tooth firmly enough onto the end of a drill bit, you can drill through aluminium or brick and the tooth ends up unmarked. Or you can heat up a tooth alongside a steel ball bearing – the ball bearing will melt long before the tooth is even slightly altered. And when you consider all the things our teeth can do, it is not surprising that they have been called the toughest little toolkit available. They can grip as powerfully as any pair of pliers; think of those trapeze artists who twirl high above the circus ring, biting on to a leather thong, with only the grip of their teeth to keep them from a fatal fall. Teeth can crush and grind as effectively as any man-made machine 50 times their size; they can cut and tear as deeply and cleanly as any chisel, saw or knife.

It is tragic therefore to think that most of us will have damaged teeth long before any other part of our bodies begins to wear out. Tough as they are, our teeth have an Achilles' heel; they are vulnerable to attack by acid. And modern food habits are precisely the last thing our teeth need. So many of our foods contain sugar, whether as a sweetener or simply a preservative, that we constantly feed the bacteria in our mouths which produce the damaging acid. Different people have different amounts of this harmful bacteria, streptococcus mutans; and that is why some of us are much more prone to tooth decay than others.

The problem is that all the strength of a tooth comes from the thin, dead, outer layer or enamel. This is made up of special crystals containing calcium minerals, which give teeth their white colour. Once we go below the enamel we come to the darker dentine, a softer living tissue which contains nerve endings. These nerve endings come from the deepest, most central living part of the tooth, the pulp. And the pulp contains the main nerves for the tooth, as well as blood vessels to supply essential nutrients, and materials to help repair minor damage.

Of course, only a small part of the tooth is visible above the gums; most of it is set deep into the gum, with roots anchoring it firmly into the jaw. Strong sinewy tissues called ligaments bind the roots firmly into the bone of the jaw and act as shock absorbers so that we can tolerate the stresses and strains we put on our teeth. The more we demand of our teeth, the more securely they will be rooted. The strong back teeth which we use for chewing and grinding have four roots, while the front teeth which specialise in slicing and cutting have only one.

When we eat, any acid produced in the mouth will trigger the production of some neutralising alkali salts in the saliva. But this is not enough to prevent a small amount of acid attack on the teeth, which dissolves some of the mineral salts from the tooth enamel. With a normal low-sugar diet, our teeth are kept reasonably clean by the constant washing they receive from the saliva. This contains enough minerals to replace the minerals in the tooth enamel which the small amount of acid dissolves out. However, when large amounts of sugar are being eaten constantly, the streptococcus mutans bacteria make much more acid than the saliva can cope with. And, as a result, holes begin to appear in the enamel which the saliva cannot repair. They become larger and deeper until the

CROSS-SECTION THROUGH A TOOTH

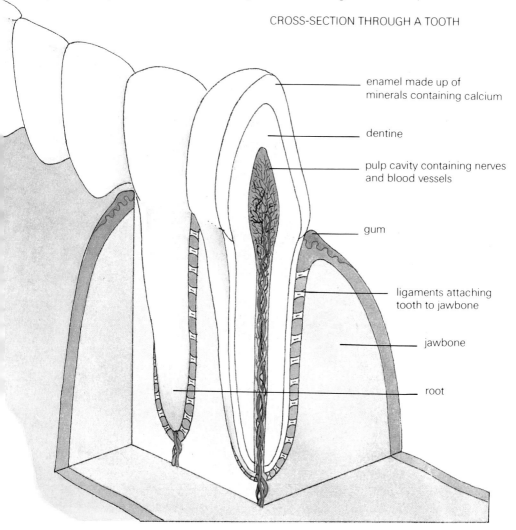

enamel made up of minerals containing calcium

dentine

pulp cavity containing nerves and blood vessels

gum

ligaments attaching tooth to jawbone

jawbone

root

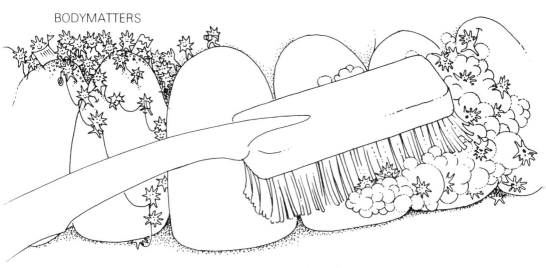

enamel is penetrated and the bacteria begin to infect the soft dentine underneath, producing the all too familiar toothache at the nerve endings, the first tell-tale sign that tooth decay has set in. The sooner it is treated the better. A filling may stop the rot, but if the damage is extensive and the infection reaches deep into the pulp, the dentist may have no alternative but to remove the tooth.

One way to help the saliva do its job of refilling holes in the enamel is to introduce special chemicals called fluorides into the mouth, either in toothpaste or in drinking water. These chemicals seem to prevent tooth decay in two ways: by filling in the holes which the saliva cannot cope with, and by strengthening the tooth enamel, so that acid finds it harder to release its minerals the next time round. This is why dentists are so keen for everyone to use a toothpaste which contains fluoride.

Perhaps the most important single thing we can all do is to keep down the amount of plaque on our teeth. Plaque is that soft spongy layer that builds up on our teeth if they are left uncleaned, and it consists of growing colonies of harmful bacteria, like streptococcus mutans. It not only causes tooth decay; it can also be respon-

Removing plaque by regular brushing prevents decay in the tooth enamel, leading to deep cavities eventually . . .

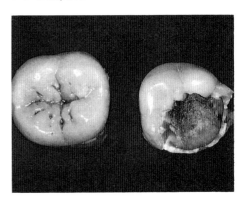

. . . which will destroy the good looks and the effectiveness of a set of perfect teeth all too easily.

sible for gum disease. This is much more widespread than most people realise; a staggering 90 per cent of us still suffer from gingivitis, or gum disease, without even realising it. If your gums bleed when you brush your teeth, or if you suffer from bad breath, you almost certainly have gingivitis. It is caused by plaque getting into little pockets between the gums and the teeth, and gradually enlarging the pockets. This causes the skin of the gums to harden and fracture easily, so that they bleed; and releases gases created by the bacteria in the plaque as they digest small food particles. These gases, in sufficient quantity, can be detected as bad breath. And if gingivitis goes unchecked for long enough, the plaque will infect a tooth from below the gum, destroying the ligaments which tie the roots into the jaw and eventually making us lose the tooth.

A sugar-free diet and regular brushing, especially in the pockets between gums and teeth, is the only answer in the long run. But so few of us are concerned about taking care of our teeth that dentists are still filling 25 000 000 teeth every year in Britain alone; and many people eventually have to put up with the inconvenience of false teeth. However good they are (and false teeth can be very lifelike and effective nowadays), they are not as tough and versatile as your original toolkit, which a little bit of care could keep in good working order all your life.

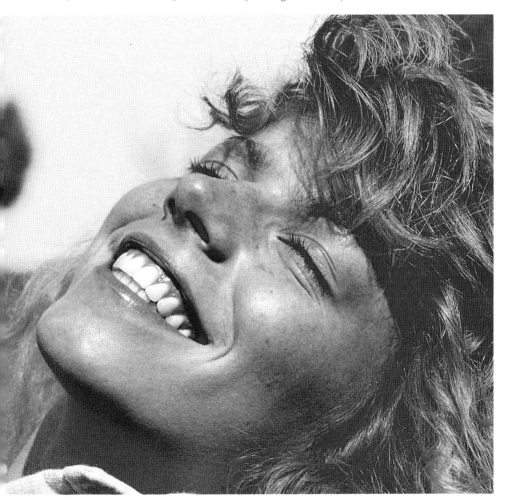

THE MUSIC ROOM ON TOP OF THE STOVE

I f we had to choose the one part of our citadel where the architect appears to have lost his marbles, it would surely have to be the larynx. Who in their right mind would want to build a main feeder tunnel into a power station, and then adapt it to incorporate a concert hall? Yet this is exactly what the larynx is – the home of our vocal cords, and the doorway to the stomach and digestive tract.

Naturally, the design is ingenious enough to help us survive such an absurd arrangement. The music room stays securely closed while we are feeding the stove; you can feel it bobbing up and down as you chew and swallow. Put your fingers lightly on your Adam's apple while you eat, and you will inevitably feel it moving. The Adam's apple is your larynx, the voice box part of your throat, which can move aside to let food go from your mouth to your stomach, and also open up to let air go to and from your lungs. When the larynx is open, the route to the stomach is closed; and you can force air from the lungs through the larynx, where it vibrates the vocal cords to produce sound. Those sounds are so carefully crafted, with the help of the nose, mouth, tongue, teeth and lips, that they can be anything from spoken language to musical notes, consciously sung words or a whole range of involuntary but emotionally expressive grunts and groans.

The main snag with the system is that, just occasionally, we do not close the music room door in time, and food goes down the wrong way; in other words, we choke. But this happens so rarely that we can, on balance, be duly impressed with the ingenious workings of the larynx, and its precious contents, the vocal cords. If you would prefer to see them spelt 'chords', that is absolutely fine; both spellings are correct, and at least one book has 'cords' in the text and 'chords' in the index! All that really matters is that we can produce musical chords by vibrating the strings or cords in our voice box.

The larynx really *is* a box, made of tough, flexible tissue called cartilage, enclosing the two vocal cords at the top of the windpipe or trachea. The larynx has a kind of lid – a sort of spring-open top like the ones on pedal bins. This is a flap of cartilage known as the epiglottis – the door to the vocal cords, which snaps shut while we eat. The actual position of the larynx changes as we grow older; when we are small babies it is so high in the mouth that we can suckle and breathe at the same time. Watch a hungry baby as it takes milk from either breast or bottle. It drinks and drinks without pausing, because the air

46

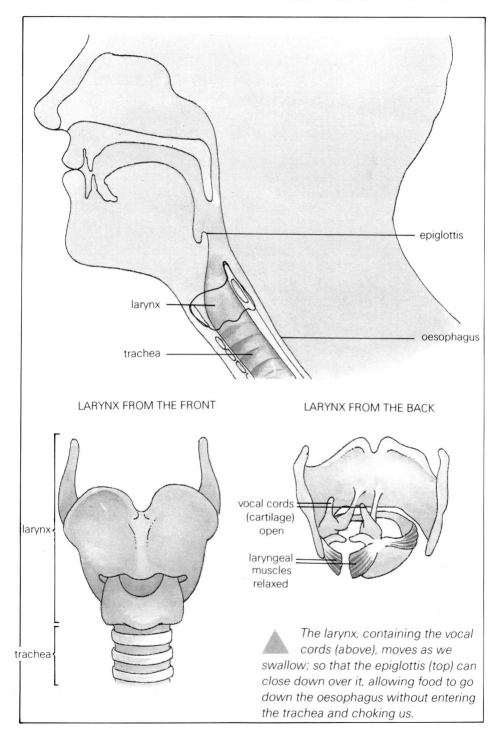

epiglottis

larynx

oesophagus

trachea

LARYNX FROM THE FRONT

LARYNX FROM THE BACK

larynx

vocal cords
(cartilage)
open

trachea

laryngeal
muscles
relaxed

The larynx, containing the vocal cords (above), moves as we swallow; so that the epiglottis (top) can close down over it, allowing food to go down the oesophagus without entering the trachea and choking us.

47

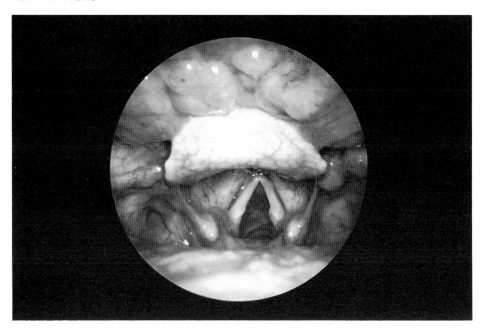

taken in through its nose can get into the trachea, while at the same time the milk taken through its mouth goes around the high larynx and down into the stomach. So, for the only time in our lives, the larynx can be open to allow air through, while it is high enough in the mouth to let food go past without entering the trachea and causing choking.

This all changes, however, because the larynx needs to settle deeper and deeper into our throats to give us the full facilities of speech and vocal range. And this deep position means that the larynx has to lie right across the pathway to the stomach, which is why we develop the complex ability to lift the larynx up and over the food we are eating, while at the same time taking a swallow to get some of it into our stomachs. This also helps to regulate how much food we take in; we swallow only a certain amount at a time, giving our mouths time to chew and break up the food to make it easier to digest. And all the

These vocal cords are at rest, wide open to allow comfortable breathing without any sounds being created.

time we are doing this, our epiglottis is instinctively kept shut – unless we insist on talking with our mouths full, when we run the risk of making ourselves choke.

This danger exists because, under normal conditions, the two vocal cords are left open with a sort of wedge-shaped gap between them. This gap allows air to pass directly into our lungs as we breathe. So any food that can squeeze by an open epiglottis finds it all too easy to slip down the windpipe towards the lungs, where it could cause no end of damage. Worst of all, if the food blocked the trachea altogether, we could soon die because no oxygen would be getting to our lungs. As an emergency procedure, we contract our muscles violently to push the food

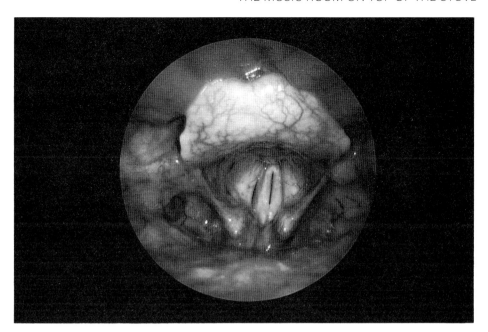

Here the cords have snapped together, so that any air breathed between them will vibrate to create sound.

back up and out of the windpipe, which is why we cough and splutter so much when we choke. The first aid treatment which can actually make the difference between life and death is to give a sudden, forceful bear hug below the ribs to drive air out of the lungs, up the trachea, and behind the food blockage, forcing it past the epiglottis and back into the mouth. Taking effective action can actually damage the muscles of the abdomen, so it is not something to try casually; it should only be used as a prompt life-saving emergency procedure.

With the danger of choking, it might seem odd that the vocal cords are naturally kept open. But the reflex action which closes the epiglottis when we eat is so quick that serious choking is a rare occurrence. And we need to have our cords open if we want to breathe and stay silent at the same time. If we want to speak, or sing, or make any sort of noise, the two cords snap shut like a couple of lift doors. Then we force air from inside the lungs to go back out into the mouth and nose cavities through the tiny gap between the closed vocal cords. As the air passes, we make the tiny muscles controlling the cords vibrate them, to produce a vibration or sound wave in the air. This is then refined by the way we make it travel through and around the mouth and nose (and even into cavities in the skull, around the cheeks and forehead) where it is amplified to an easily heard level.

It is very similar to the way a musician varies sounds in a wind instrument. Imagine, say, the twisting coils and turns of the French horn as the cavities in our nose and mouth. We can vary the shape and resonance of the horn by pressing the valves closed or leaving them open; and the various combinations of open and closed valves create a whole range of notes. In the same way, the position of the tongue, lips and teeth can refine the sound wave we force through our vocal cords. As soon as we forgo the use of even one of these refining possibilities, we noticeably restrict our vocal talents. Try saying the famous ventriloquist's challenge, 'bottle of beer' without moving your lips and without making the words sound like 'gottle of geer'!

The reason you find it so hard is that the lips are used to put a final distinctive touch to a 'b' sound. This involves closing them and then letting the emerging sound wave force them apart as it leaves the mouth. We need a similar finish to 'p' and 'm' sounds; but in these cases the sound waves have been subtly prepared in a different way before they reach the lips. Make 'b', 'p' and 'm' sounds for yourself, and see if you can feel what is going on in your mouth to make the sounds different. If the differences are just too subtle for you to detect, try making 't' and 'k' sounds. They both depend on the tongue rising up to the palate, or roof of the mouth, and then being lowered as the sound wave moves through; but in the case of 'k' it touches the palate near the back, and with 't' it is right behind the teeth at the front.

The ventriloquist of course finds clever ways round the most obvious lip movements when making sounds; and it certainly isn't easy. Try touching the back of the palate with the tip of your tongue, and then making any of the five sounds we have just tried. You will be lucky to distinguish between the strangulated noises which result, and you will probably feel like choking if you try too hard to get the tongue really far back. That is because the nerve endings at the back of the mouth sense that there is something in the way which you cannot or will not swallow, and so they trigger what is known as the gagging reflex to push back out of the mouth whatever is lodged in this sensitive position. It is just part of the whole complex nerve and muscle reaction which makes us throw up when we want to get something unpleasant or poisonous out of our throats and stomachs.

But to get back to the more comfortable and tasteful subject of our vocal abilities. Besides having so many variations in the way we shape sounds in our mouth and nose, we can also vary the speed at which the vocal cords vibrate, and the force with which air is pushed past them. This allows us to produce higher or lower notes, and louder or softer sounds. Opera singers are as dependent as athletes on regular training, because they need to develop control of the diaphragm (a muscular part of the abdomen which expels air from the lungs) as well as the tiny muscles controlling the vocal cords and the whole range of tongue, lip and palate positions. But the two tiny vocal cords are crucial to producing a smooth sound. When they become infected, they swell and cannot close together properly, or vibrate smoothly – which is why you lose your voice, or it sounds hoarse and weak, when you have a throat infection.

When you reflect on how much this tiny box of cartilage does for you, it is worth taking good care of it. The music room may well be in a bizarre position on top of the stove, but with the minimum of good maintenance it will continue to provide more sound variations than you could ever hope to hear from any man-made musical instrument.

50

FUELLING
THE SYSTEM

You may not have thought of it before, but the truth is that you are rather like a doughnut. Or, to be more accurate, a 'donut', because that is how the Americans spell it, and Americans make doughnuts with holes through the middle. But don't worry – you are not alone; we are all built this way, with a long tubular hole running right through us, from the mouth at the top to the – well, to the bottom! And this hole through the middle enables us to fuel our whole living system, from anything that we pass through it.

The tube (known as the digestive tract) is not quite as empty as the usual sort of hole, since all the way along it are a number of sphincters. These are rings of muscle which contract to form a tight seal – a bit like a rubber band around the neck of a polythene bag. We open and close the sphincters so that whatever we take into our mouths can be passed from one part of the tube to the next during the digestive process. There are sphincters, for instance, at either end of the part of the tube we call the stomach, so that we can keep food inside it for hours. We need to compartmentalise the digestive tract with these sphincters because anything we eat gets processed, a stage at a time, as it passes through. It is transformed from the fruit, meat and vegetables we first taste and chew into a chemical purée from which we extract valuable fuels for our body, leaving unwanted materials as waste products which we dispose of when we open the anal sphincter.

Since every living cell in our bodies needs constant refuelling to do its job properly, it is obviously vital to take in the right amount of exactly the right kinds of food. This is why we have appetites which not only tell us that we are hungry, but also discriminate between one kind of food

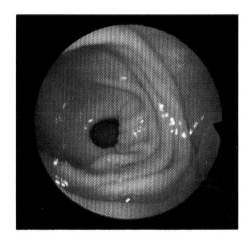

▲ *This sphincter can close to seal off the bottom end of the stomach where it continues into the duodenum.*

and another. Imagine yourself on two different holidays, about to order lunch. After a morning spent skiing, you might well prefer the hot beef goulash and fried potatoes; while after lazing on a Mediterranean beach it would probably be fish and salad. The high proportion of fat in the first meal is needed to replenish the supply which has been used up on the slopes both by energetic activity and the need to keep warm; while the second meal offers low fat and high water content, ideal after a morning doing nothing but sunbathing, when the main thing the body needs to replenish is the water lost in perspiration as it kept cool.

Once our brains have received the message that we are hungry and in need of a certain kind of food, any hint that the required food is in reach triggers the beginning of the digestive process. Given that we have only the slightest need for them, the smell of fried onions or the sight of a succulent steak, for example, will cause our mouths to water; and this is a vital first step if we are to eat anything. Try challenging a friend to see who can be the first to eat three dry cream crackers without a drink or anything else. If you can manage more than two, you are either amazingly hungry with a mouth positively brimming with water, or your masochistic competitive spirit is exceptional! The digestive system wants a lot of saliva (the water in your mouth) to lubricate the food and help it on its way down the gullet, but the cream crackers simply absorb it like blotting paper.

Once the combination of appetite and saliva have got food into your mouth, where it can be cut and chewed a little to help it on its way past your larynx, you lose interest in what happens from here on in. Mercifully so, because the food is going to spend another 4 hours being processed, and you will want to get on with other things without having to think continually of steak and onions! The 16 or so inches of tube after the larynx is known as the oesophagus, and muscles in the oesophagus quickly manhandle the incoming food to the first sphincter, at the top of the stomach. It does not just fall there by gravity; so you can eat lying down or even the wrong way up if you really want to!

The oesophagus is a fairly stiff and narrow part of the digestive tract compared with the stomach, which is more of a soft-sided bag between the two sphincters at either end. Most people think of the stomach as the most significant part of the digestive system, and therefore assume that most of the valuable fuels we need are passed into the body from here. But in fact very little can go from the stomach into the body – only alcohol and drugs like aspirin. The prime task of the stomach is to act exactly like a mechanical food mixer in the kitchen; it breaks down the food into tiny bits and thoroughly mixes fragments of steak, chips and onions with the peaches and cream that followed. Of course it does not use metal blades to grind the food; instead it breaks everything down with a powerful acid and chemicals called enzymes.

As food enters the stomach, it triggers the production of yet another chemical, a hormone called gastrin. This hormone effectively controls the whole working of the stomach. First of all, cells in the stomach wall produce hydrochloric acid to mix in with the food, killing off any harmful bacteria and beginning to break it down. Then the enzymes are added. They thrive in the acid environment of the stomach and each type of enzyme goes to work processing particular food substances. Perhaps the most important is pepsin, an enzyme which acts a bit like specialist scissors, seeking out proteins in the food and cutting them up into tiny pieces to make them more manageable further down the digestive tract.

The acid in the stomach has to be very strong to do its job; and if it burns the stomach wall, creating a gastric ulcer, you can certainly feel its corrosive power. Normally the stomach handles the acid without pain because its lining produces a thick slimy mucus to protect itself. This mucus contains bicarbonates, which are of course alkaline, thus neutralising any acid which attempts to corrode the

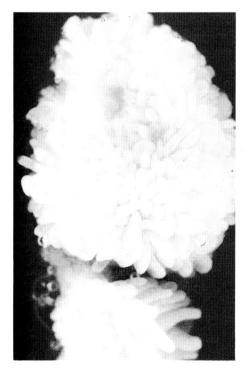

Millions of these finger-like structures line the small intestine so that different foods can be absorbed and taken to where they are needed.

stomach wall. If the system fails, then painful ulcers can result. Other, much less painful, problems are caused by the acid leaking out through the sphincters without being neutralised. At the entrance to the stomach, acid can burn the wall of the oesophagus, producing the typical symptoms of indigestion and heartburn.

After 4 hours in the stomach, the food is ready for further processing, but still not ready to release its fuel supply into the body. In the next 10 inches of the digestive tract (a sharp bend called the duodenum), it is the turn of the fats and the carbohydrates to be cut into tiny pieces. First of all, bile is released from the liver and stored in the gall bladder, ready to work on the fats. As soon as the broken-down food mixture enters the duodenum, the bile is squeezed in through the bile duct to join it. The bile acts in a similar way to detergent, reducing the lumps of fat to tiny droplets that are easily mixed in with the rest of the liquids in the digestive tract. The next duct along the duodenum brings in a fluid containing three enzymes from the pancreas: trypsin which continues the work of the pepsin in cutting up the proteins, lipase which carries on with breaking down the fats, and amylase which gets going on the carbohydrates.

By now the food travelling along the digestive tract will have become a kind of liquid emulsion, its bulk significantly increased by all the juices which have been added along the way: saliva to start with, then a good litre of stomach juices, as well as the bile and enzyme solution in the duodenum. And all that has been shed are aspirins and alcohol. So, not surprisingly, in the next part of the tract (the small intestine) the real absorption begins. This 19-foot-long coiled tube contains a mass of finger-like structures which wave like the antennae on a sea anemone, ready to catch the bits of food as they float past. Each of these special 'fishermen' is covered in a series of specially shaped 'slots' through which only one particular type of fuel can be 'posted'. One set of slots link up with the lymphatic system (a network of glands which distribute the fats around the body); the others take in the proteins and carbohydrates and pass them into the bloodstream through tiny blood vessels. Since the food has to be so microscopically small to be absorbed, it is hardly surprising that there is a surface area of some 10 square yards packed into the small intestine.

Finally, what is left of the food enters the large intestine. This is really a 7-foot-long waste processing plant, but even here we absorb fuels for the body, in particular some disease-fighting fatty acids from the fibrous content of plants we have eaten. There are several folds of tissue which squeeze water out of the waste matter and transfer it to the kidneys via the bloodstream. Here it can be cleansed and recycled, except for a small amount which is used to flush the kidneys clean before being expelled as urine. Meanwhile the much drier bulk of the waste in the large intestine is being digested by bacteria to produce those useful fatty acids and package the waste ready for disposal.

So the full 30 feet of our guts is quite an active place, absorbing around 400 grams of assorted fuels every day to keep us going. That may not sound much, but in the process each of us has had to produce and recycle some 6 litres of fluid; and perhaps to our embarrassment when in public places we also need to release a staggering 2 litres of gas by-products from the work of the bacteria in the large intestine!

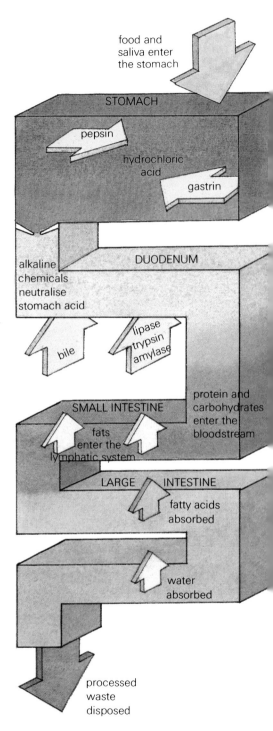

food and saliva enter the stomach

STOMACH

pepsin

hydrochloric acid

gastrin

alkaline chemicals neutralise stomach acid

DUODENUM

lipase
trypsin
amylase

bile

SMALL INTESTINE

fats enter the lymphatic system

protein and carbohydrates enter the bloodstream

LARGE INTESTINE

fatty acids absorbed

water absorbed

processed waste disposed

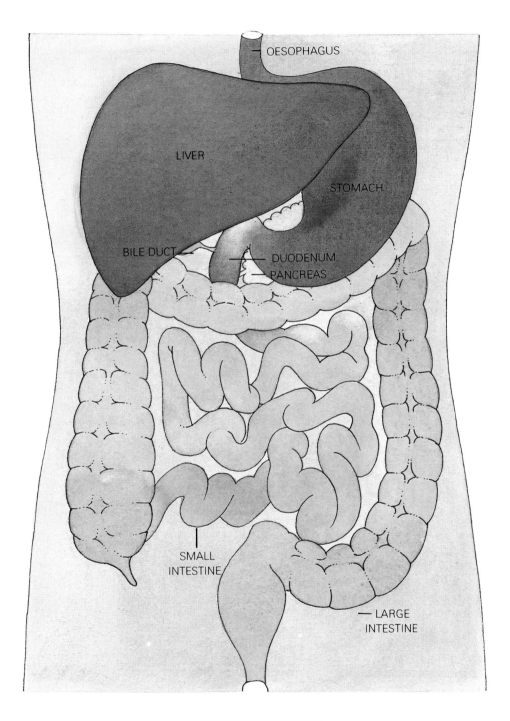

OESOPHAGUS

LIVER

STOMACH

BILE DUCT

DUODENUM
PANCREAS

SMALL
INTESTINE

LARGE
INTESTINE

THE DIGESTIVE SYSTEM

SELF-FILLING GAS TANKS

The lungs hold a lot of surprises for anyone who is not entirely familiar with the way our bodies work. For a start, how much air would you think you could get into them? Most people would guess at a couple of milk bottles full on either side of the chest, but they would be nowhere near correct. Between them, our lungs can manage around nine whole milk bottles full of air – a massive 5 litres in all. But we only breathe a fraction of that under normal circumstances. If we are not running for our lives, a typical breathing pattern would be to inhale about half a litre of fresh air – including virtually no carbon dioxide and over 20 per cent oxygen; and then to exhale about half a litre of spent gases – including 4 per cent carbon dioxide and 16 per cent oxygen. The rest of the air we breathe is virtually unaffected; 78 per cent nitrogen is breathed in and 78 per cent gets breathed out.

But why does the proportion of oxygen and carbon dioxide change, and why do we use such a small fraction of the huge space in our lungs? It is easiest to deal with the question of capacity first. After allowing for the half litre involved in regular breathing, the rest of our 5 litres is simply spare capacity, which we call on when in dire straits – if the lungs are damaged or infected, or when we need to exert ourselves to cope with some immediate crisis. The proportion of the two gases changes because the process of breathing actually extracts some oxygen from the air we breathe in for our body to use. We then exchange the oxygen for carbon dioxide, which has been built up by the body using oxygen from earlier breaths.

Every living cell in the body needs to combine food and oxygen to release energy, otherwise we would not be able to keep going! And our cells receive food and oxygen from the same transport system – the blood flowing all round the body like a non-stop goods train. The cells produce carbon dioxide as a waste product when combining the two fuels, food and oxygen. And when any one part of the body unloads the 'goods train', in particular when it takes oxygen molecules from red blood cells, it immediately refills some of the empty spaces left in the cells by loading them with carbon dioxide molecules. A lot more carbon dioxide is simply transported in the liquid part of the blood, called the plasma. The 'train' continues its journey all round the body until eventually the blood arrives back at the

▶ *A resin cast of the complex and delicate branches of a pair of human lungs.*

56

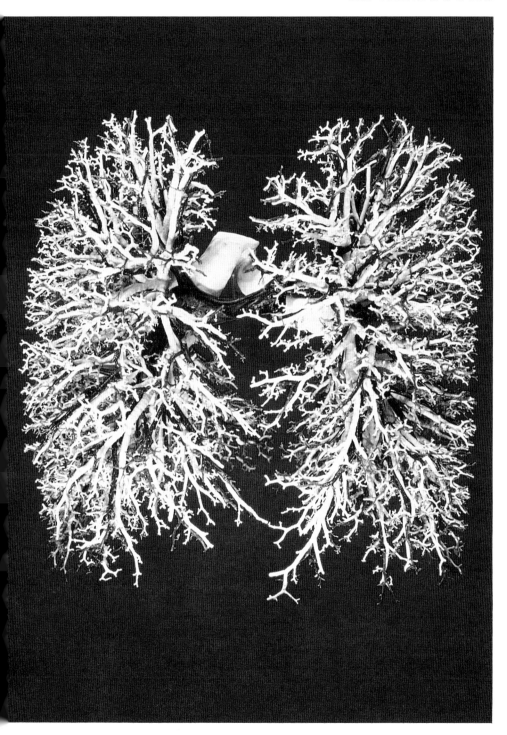

lungs again. Here the carbon dioxide is unloaded, to be breathed out; and newly inhaled oxygen is loaded back into the red blood cells for distribution around the body once more.

In order to keep up this constant gas exchange, our lungs need to load and unload millions of red blood cells in every breath. And this is where the next surprise comes in. To accommodate all the required exchange points, the lungs need an enormous surface area – in fact roughly 100 square metres (in other words, the size of a wall-to-wall carpet in an average bedroom!). And in order to cram all that surface area into our chests, the lungs are designed in an ingenious and amazingly beautiful way. They are not merely balloon-like bags, as many people assume; they are more like delicate hollow trees.

The trunks of the two trees join the trachea, or windpipe, roughly 6 to 9 inches below your larynx. These hollow tubes are called the bronchi; and if you get asthma they can contract in spasms, preventing air getting in or out of the lungs. They also get clogged up with mucus (and so partially closed) if we get bronchitis, which is why our breathing becomes so difficult then. These bronchi branch off from the trachea to the left and the right of the chest cavity, and then divide into smaller and smaller branches, spreading out like the branches of a chestnut tree, until the whole chest cavity is completely filled with an amazing network of narrower and narrower tubes. And it is right at the ends of the narrowest of these tubes that the gas exchanges take place.

The tiny air sacs at the ends of these tubes are called alveoli; and though tiny, they are immensely sophisticated. They secrete a fluid which traps molecules of oxygen as they arrive, so the oxygen flows all over the inside wall of the sac. The oxygen can then pass through this wall, still carried in the fluid, rather like coffee and water passing through a filter in a coffee machine. The outside of the alveoli is surrounded by tiny thin-walled blood vessels;

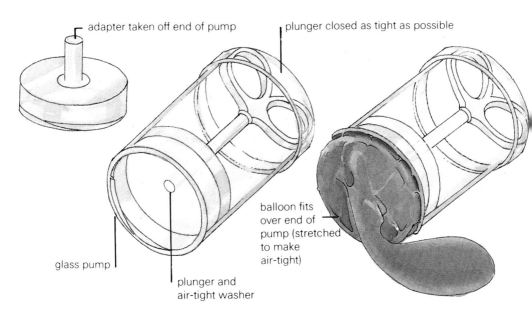

adapter taken off end of pump

plunger closed as tight as possible

glass pump

plunger and air-tight washer

balloon fits over end of pump (stretched to make air-tight)

and once again, the oxygen-bearing fluid can pass through the walls and into the blood. There it is picked up by haemoglobin, a special chemical in the red blood cells, and taken off around the blood system to all parts of the body.

Just the reverse happens with the carbon dioxide. It is transferred from haemoglobin or the plasma, through the walls of the blood vessels, through the walls of the alveoli, and into the air sacs. From there, it is taken away the next time we breathe out, along the branches of the lung to the bronchi and then out up the trachea.

And this leads us to the lungs' last surprise. Most people assume that the air we breathe in is somehow pumped into us by the lungs, and then let out again by the lungs when we breathe out. The surprise is that the lungs do not 'do' anything at all; they are rather like sponges in the sense that they soak up air when allowed to expand, and squeeze it out again when squashed down. But in fact the lungs are really sponges in reverse. Their natural elasticity means that, left to their own devices, they would shrink inwards like a collapsed balloon; in other words, they would be like a tightly squeezed sponge. But there is a vacuum between the lungs and the chest wall, and at the bottom of the chest there is a huge muscular part of the wall called the diaphragm. When we breathe in, the diaphragm pulls down, the vacuum stretches the lungs open, and they suck in air to fill the hollow tubes. We allow sufficient time for the gas exchange to take place, and then we relax the diaphragm. The elastic lungs shrink back to their original size, expelling the gases inside them at the same time; and we breathe out.

You can see the principle for yourself quite easily if you do a little experiment with a wide football pump. Take the nozzle and adapter off the end of the pump and, with the plunger fully compressed, insert a balloon. Stretch the neck of the balloon around the open end of the pump.

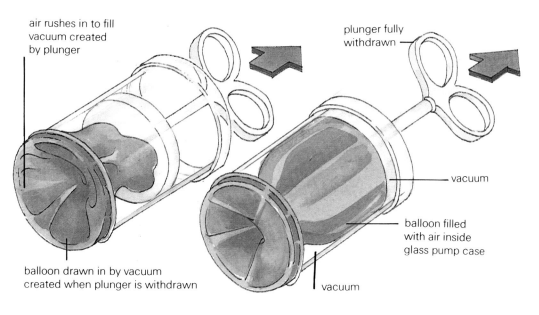

air rushes in to fill vacuum created by plunger

plunger fully withdrawn

vacuum

balloon filled with air inside glass pump case

balloon drawn in by vacuum created when plunger is withdrawn

vacuum

If you now pull the plunger out, it will be like the diaphragm lowering, and you will see the balloon being sucked inwards and stretching – just like a lung filling with air. This self-filling gas tank will stay full until you release the plunger and the balloon shrinks back, expelling the air and getting ready to fill itself once more.

Don't worry if you haven't got a wide enough pump to get a balloon inside it; if you can follow the principle you should be able to work out what is happening in your own body. If you have ever been 'winded', you will know all about it; a nasty blow below the waist can make the muscles there contract involuntarily, so the diaphragm stops working for a few seconds. As you wait helplessly for the muscles to relax and the lungs to start filling again, you will certainly be aware that the self-filling mechanism in your gas tanks has been temporarily stopped!

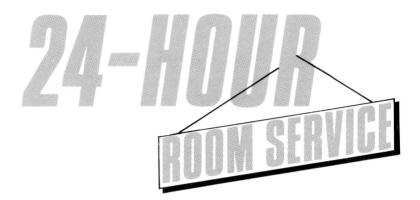

In exploring our citadel from top to bottom, we have reached halfway without taking much notice of one or two things that do not simply occupy part of the body, but are present literally everywhere. Admittedly, we had a good look at nerves on our way round the head; but we have skipped over skin and bone, muscles and blood. So we might as well take a quick look at each of them, before we dash off down our arms to explore the workings of our hands.

In fact we have already had a reasonable look at the blood, the non-stop goods train which provides every part of our bodies with 24-hour room service. We could not have appreciated the way our guts and lungs work without mentioning it. And as we all know, the reason for the non-stop nature of the blood is that it is pumped around the body by one huge central muscle – the heart. But there are a few other things about the blood system which are perhaps not quite so obvious.

The blood of course travels away from the heart, pushed along through wide strong arteries, and then finds its way into thinner and thinner blood vessels called capillaries.

By the time it has reached these delicate thin tubes at every point in the body, the blood is a long way from the initial powerful driving force of the heart, so the pumping action is no longer very strong. This is fortunate because the delicate capillaries might burst if more forceful surges of blood were driven into them. However, it means that as the blood flows back towards the heart, away from the capillaries and into larger and larger veins, there is less and less force to push it along. So our veins contain a series of one-way valves to make sure that the blood does not run backwards, and keeps going in the right direction. In addition, muscles all around the veins push the blood along by contracting and relaxing in turn.

Incidentally, if you find it hard to believe that any part of the blood system could be very far away from the heart, perhaps you should try to work out just how long all the blood vessels in a single, average-sized, adult body would be if we joined them up end to end. There are a staggering 96 500 kilometres of them – enough to stretch comfortably twice round the world!

You may not normally be able to see how your blood circulation works; but you can see it indirectly if you are unfortunate enough to cut yourself badly. If you have bright scarlet blood coming out of the wound in surges, you need to close the wound firmly and quickly because you

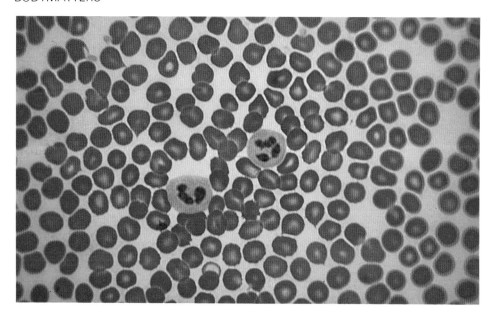

have severed an artery. The surges are the pumping of the heart behind the blood, and the bright red colour shows that the blood is full of oxygen on its way to help fuel all parts of the body. If the blood is a darker, more purply colour, and it flows steadily, then you will have cut a vein. With most minor cuts, of course, you only damage small capillaries near the skin's surface.

The cuts soon heal because the blood carries a repair kit with it wherever it goes. As well as the oxygen-carrying red blood cells, it contains white blood cells which are designed to fight unwanted viruses and bacteria. The white blood cells fight diseases as well as rushing to the site of a wound where they start disinfecting the area ready for healing to take place. At the same time, the blood contains platelets and special chemicals called clotting factors which work together to stop the blood flowing out of the wound, seal it up, and let healing continue under a protective scab. The clotting factors react to a

You can see just two white blood cells amongst a mass of red blood cells in this sample of blood, magnified over 200 times.

This simplified plan of the circulation represents nearly 100 000 kilometres of blood vessels.

DETAIL OF ARTERIES DIVIDING INTO CAPILLARIES

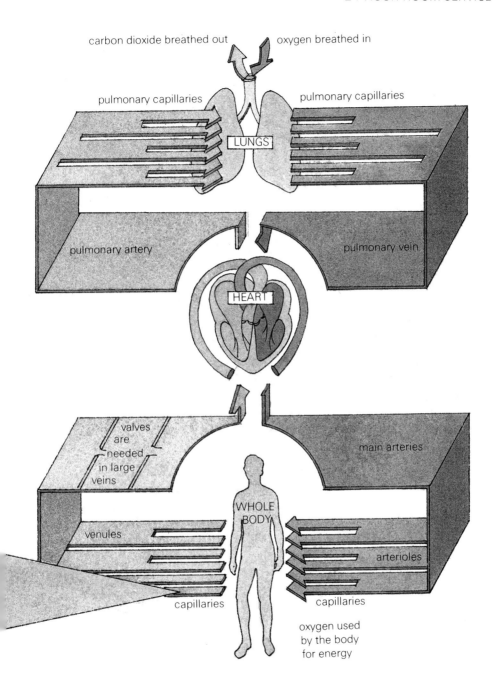

THE CIRCULATORY SYSTEM

chemical released by the cut cells in the wound, and as each triggers the next in a chain reaction, a series of protein strands called fibrin are made. They criss-cross each other to form a kind of lattice pattern. At the same time, the platelets become 'sticky' and fill in the gaps in the latticework created by the fibrin, forming a clot.

So blood contains a lot of different ingredients. The platelets, clotting factors, white and red blood cells are all solid. The liquid part of the blood is called plasma – it is clear and yellowish, and contains 90 per cent water. Blood is red because of the red cells, which form about half its bulk. There are 600 red cells for every white cell, and there are fewer platelets than white cells.

The plasma also contains all the food and waste products which the blood delivers and collects on its way around the body, as well as the clotting factors and other essential chemicals needed to keep the blood flowing efficiently. These chemicals have to be compatible with the red cells in the blood, or the blood could start to clot anywhere in the system, with dire consequences. That is why our blood groups are clearly identified before we are given a blood transfusion in an emergency. On the outside of the red blood cells are about 200 different tiny proteins, called antigens. We all have different combinations, according to what we have inherited from our parents; but for most blood grouping purposes we only need to examine three or four of them.

The first thing to test for are the 'A' and 'B' antigens. If you have neither of them on your red cells, you will be in the most common blood group, 'O'. If you have both of them, you will be 'AB'. And if you only have one of them, you will be either 'A' or 'B' accordingly. Another antigen test decides whether you are rhesus positive or negative. 'Rh+' is far more common than 'Rh−', but it is important to identify the few 'Rh−' patients because it could prove fatal if they were given 'Rh+' blood. Similarly, you have to be careful which blood you give to 'A's, 'B's and 'O's.

This is because of the way the white cells work to combat foreign invaders. They help produce special chemicals called antibodies, which fit onto antigens on an invading virus, for example, and then disable and destroy it. The antibodies then remain in the plasma, ready to deal with the invaders if ever they attack the body again. Clearly, each blood group would destroy itself if we could make and carry antibodies in our plasma which could latch onto the antigens on our own red blood cells.

Because of all the restrictions on the type of blood which can be given to each recipient, it is vital that the National Blood Transfusion Service collects and stores enough blood of all types in case of emergency. People die if they lose so much blood that the non-stop delivery of food and oxygen around the body cannot continue. The few minutes it takes for you to give blood could save a life.

POWER UNITS

All the energy created from the way our cells combine food and oxygen has to be harnessed to allow us to do things. And the power units which make the most direct use of energy are our muscles. Some muscles are always at work, keeping our heart beating or the digestive tract in operation, for instance; but over 600 of them (making up over a third of our body weight) are directly under the control of our willpower. They have to work in pairs because they can only exert force by contracting. For example, if you want to point to something and then return your arm to its original

MUSCLE ACTION
IN THE ARM

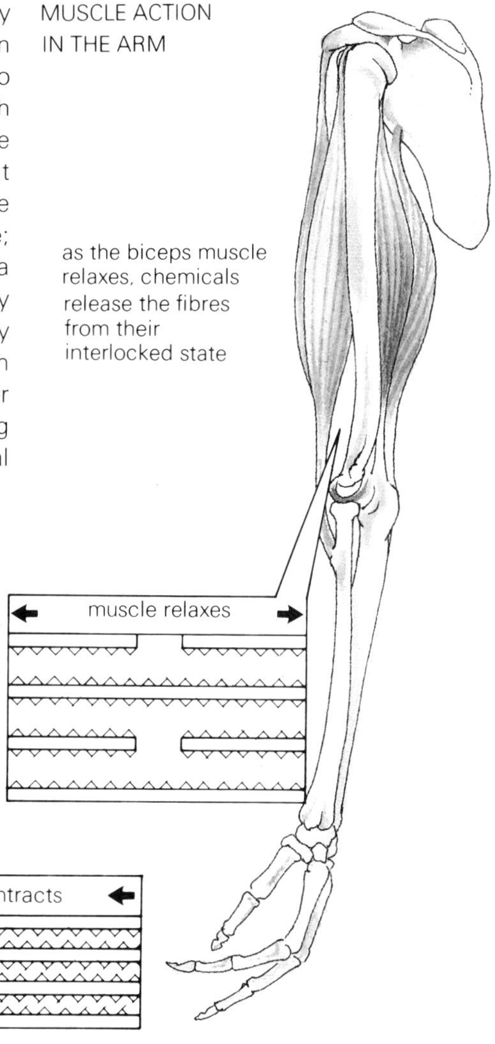

as the biceps muscle relaxes, chemicals release the fibres from their interlocked state

muscle relaxes

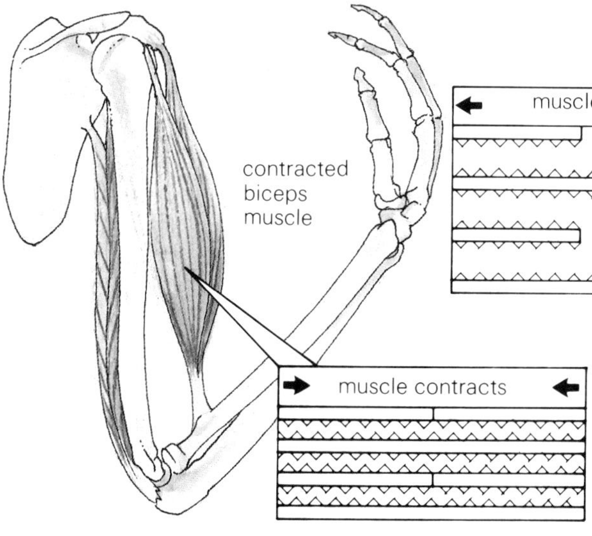

contracted
biceps
muscle

muscle contracts

position, one set of muscles contracts to move your arm forward; then, as those muscles relax, the partner set contracts to move the arm back again.

If you look at muscles under a microscope, you can see that they are actually bundles of long fibres. And when we need to move an arm or lift an object, it is those fibres which have to contract. Chemical messages from the brain travel down the appropriate nerves (through a chain of chemical reactions) to 'tell' the muscle fibres to go into action. The chain of chemical reactions ends when calcium is released to the tiny protein filaments which make up the fibres. Some of the protein, called myosin, is a bit like a team of tug-of-war athletes in search of a rope. And another protein, called actin, is rather like the rope, but it is all covered up and impossible to grip.

The arrival of the calcium at the actin uncovers some good gripping places on the rope; and the myosin latches onto these points and pulls the rope in as far as it can. (The calcium also activates the myosin, incidentally, so that it uses energy to latch on and pull.) Because the myosin cannot move backwards like a real tug-of-war team, each bit of it transfers its grip to a point a bit higher up the rope and continues to pull the actin in. While one bit of myosin is pulling, another is changing its grip; and so the actin is continually pulled in until the muscle is fully contracted. As we relax the muscle, the calcium is removed, the myosin lets go, and the actin covers up its grippable points, so that it can smoothly slide back to its starting position. And, of course, all this happens in a fraction of a second.

That probably sounds sophisticated enough, but it is really only half of the story. In each muscle there are two kinds of fibre; fast-twitch and slow-twitch. You can see the difference in a roast turkey! The white breast meat is full of fast-twitch fibres, while the darker leg meat contains a lot of slow-twitch fibres. The fast fibres are excellent for short bursts of explosive activity, like flapping a turkey's wings or driving a sprinter over 100 metres in less than 10 seconds. The slow fibres use energy much more economically, and so they can keep a turkey or a long-distance

Body-builders develop spectacular muscles – but not everyone wants this type of physique.

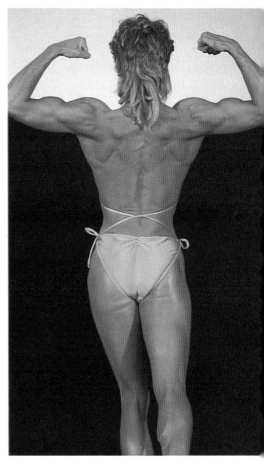

athlete running without stopping for a long period of time.

Repeated use of any muscles will of course develop them, but the slow-twitch and fast-twitch fibres respond differently to training. A sprinter, who will have inherited from his or her parents a high proportion of fast fibres in the leg muscles, will work in a series of repeated short bursts of intense activity, because this will increase the number of filaments in his or her muscle fibres. This gives more power without reducing the proportion of fast fibres in the muscles. A long-distance runner, who has inherited a relatively high proportion of slow fibres in the leg muscles, will train with long sustained runs. This seems to increase the number of blood vessels reaching the fibres, allowing more oxygen to get to them and so fuelling their energy needs more efficiently.

In the end, you are stuck with the kind of muscle you have inherited. You will not become an Olympic athlete unless the basic potential is there to start with. But you can get a lot more out of your power units by exercising, and 7-stone weaklings *can* become showcases for rippling muscles – if they really want to!

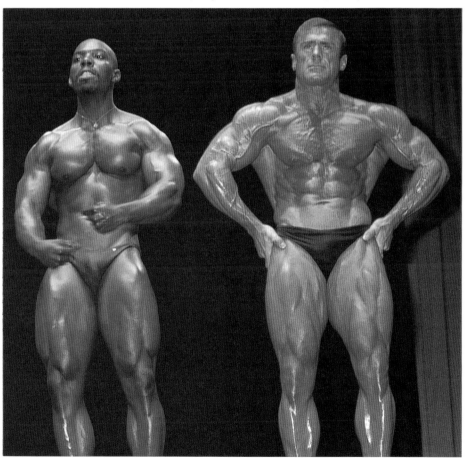

A STRONG AND FLEXIBLE FRAMEWORK

Dem bones, dem bones, dem dry bones . . .' Why does this Negro spiritual say our bones are dry? They will eventually dry out of course, when we are dead and buried, but the clothes horse on which we hang our living bodies is just as much alive (and growing and changing) as any other cells and tissues. Bones contain bone marrow and blood vessels, cartilage and collagen; and they have to be alive and able to grow, or babies would never get any bigger.

They also have to be amazingly strong, yet light and thin. We would be terribly

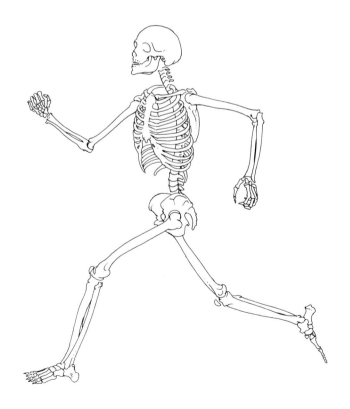

slow movers, like tortoises, if we had a heavy skeleton. Tortoises have evolved with an 'outside' skeleton, which surrounds and protects them. So instead of running away from danger, they simply stand still and draw themselves into their skeletons, because that is what a tortoise shell is – the framework on which a tortoise body is built. We evolved like many other animals with an 'inside' skeleton, so we have no outer protection from danger, but instead the ability to outwit an attacker and run! A lightweight skeleton is vital for efficient running, but it also has to be strong enough to support the loads our muscles can lift and carry. The heaviest weight known to have been lifted by a man is over 2¾ tonnes!

In order to be light but strong, our bones are a combination of a rubbery substance called collagen (which gives them enough flexibility to absorb shock when stressed) and a stiffening, more brittle mixture of mineral salts, predominantly calcium. But the real weight saving comes from their structure. They are all hollow – even thin flat bones like the skull. And the outer part of each bone is itself made up of masses of hollow tubes.

You can prove for yourself how strong a hollow tube is by balancing a glass of water on a £5 note. Just roll the note into a tube about three-quarters of an inch in diameter, stand it on end, keeping it rolled up between your fingers, and carefully position the full glass on top of it. The weight of the glass will stop the note unfurling, and you will be able to let go

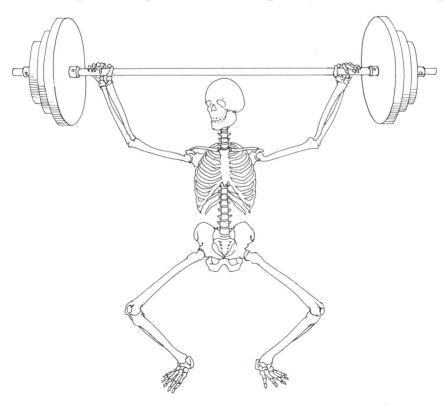

69

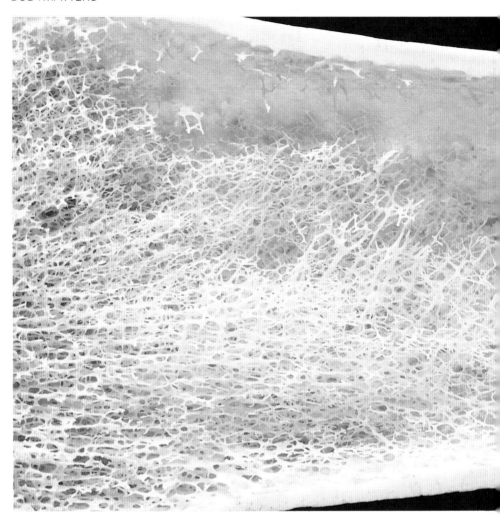

and see that the rolled note really does support it.

The pattern of a tube made up of little tubes works well for the 'stem' part of our stick-like long bones, such as those in our arms, legs, and even fingers and ribs. But the structure has to be adapted at the very ends of those bones, where they are shaped in complicated ways to join other bones, as at the ankle, hip, wrist and shoulder. The same adaptation is needed for non-tubular bones, such as the skull, pelvis and shoulder blade. A cross-section of any of these bones would reveal a typical pattern – an elaborate latticework rather like the inside of a cathedral roof – in which lines of bone act as rafters interwoven to create hollow vaults and arches cleverly shaped to brace against the loads that will be put on them.

The net result is that we have over 200 strong hollow bones in our bodies, and yet a typical adult skeleton weighs less than 9 pounds. And all those hollow spaces are

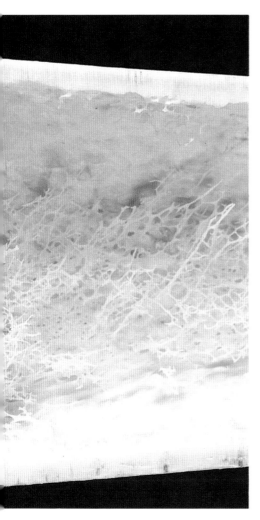

The honeycomb interior of the bone gives it lightness and strength, as well as leaving space for the production of blood cells.

we are fighting off an infection, then it will be the white cells which are in the greatest demand.

The blood's ingredients are produced when some of the cells in the bone divide and multiply. Instead of just reproducing themselves, these cells also produce a blood ingredient at the same time, before getting on with their own work within the bone. Bone cells can have a variety of specialist tasks, all connected with keeping the bone alive and well. Perhaps most interesting of all are the cells which repair broken bones and make bones grow. First of all, there are 'destroyer' cells which break down and remove any debris, such as splinters of broken bone after a fracture. They can also eat their way into new collagen, usually in the form of cartilage, to carve out the latticework pattern in the bones. Then there are the 'builder' cells, which make new mineralised bone in the spaces left for them by the 'destroyer' cells.

When we break a bone, the 'builder' cells quickly put up a kind of temporary scaffolding around the fracture, so that the slower process of restructuring the bone can go on in a protected environment. For quite a while the limb will feel bigger than it should be at the point of repair because of this 'scaffolding' around the bone, and when the fracture is eventually healed the 'destroyer' cells will demolish the 'scaffolding'.

The same cells work together to make our bones grow. There are bands of cartilage in each bone which, if left to their own devices, would simply expand stead-

not wasted either. Inside our bones there is a jelly-like bone marrow which manufactures the ingredients of our blood: red and white cells and platelets. Blood vessels which run into the bones carry the new ingredients into the bloodstream, as well as somehow conveying messages to the bone marrow to let it know what is in short supply. If we have a severe cut, we want more platelets to help form a clot; if we are anaemic, or we have just donated blood, we will be short of red cells; and if

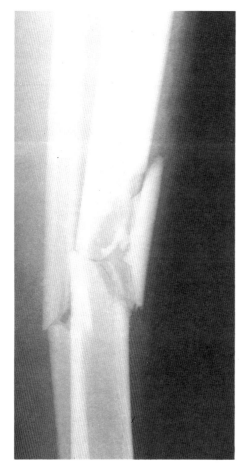
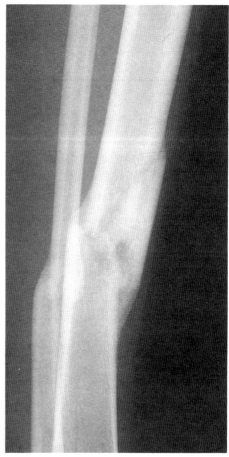

ily until we reached full adult size. But of course this would leave us with flexible rubbery bones, so the 'destroyer' cells make spaces in the cartilage for the 'builder' cells to come in and add minerals, creating new stiff, hard bone.

This means that at the beginning of our lives, when we want to grow fast, our bones contain a lot of flexible collagen and unconverted cartilage, which is why children can get so-called 'greenstick' fractures – the bone is so flexible that it only cracks halfway across and then bends. And the reverse is true in old age. We have long since stopped wanting our

These two X-rays show how a bone repairs itself. By the time of the second X-ray, 'builder' cells have started to construct a 'scaffold' around the fracture.

bones to grow, so the maximum possible amount of conversion has been completed, leaving our bones at their least flexible. Indeed, if the collagen content of the bones gets reduced too much, then old people can develop quite brittle bones, making them more vulnerable to fractures if they fall.

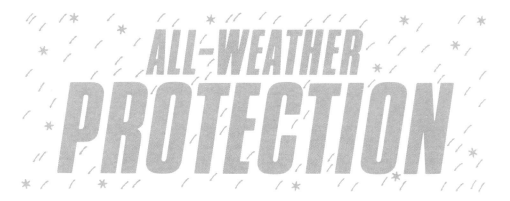

ALL-WEATHER PROTECTION

If you were not expecting to discover that our bones were full of life, then brace yourself for another surprise. The outside of our bodies is in fact dead. The surface of the skin is made up of dead cells, waiting to flake off and become minute particles drifting slowly to the ground, which is why 80 per cent of household dust is actually dead skin!

It is all in a good cause, however, because this layer of dead cells is the essential top coating of a very sophisticated all-weather protection system. Besides being a big bag in which to carry all the bits in our bodies, the skin is designed to keep us warm in the cold, and let us cool down when we are too hot. The average person's skin would cover an area of 18 square feet if it was spread out flat, and weigh around 10 pounds – only slightly more than your skeleton.

If you could examine a magnified cross-section of the skin, you would see what a complicated kind of wrapping paper it really is.

The innermost part of the skin, or dermis, is packed full of fat cells, hair follicles and glands which pump out sweat and other fluids, including chemicals called pheromones which are supposed to attract the opposite sex. There are nerves and blood vessels of course, to carry messages and to supply food and oxygen to all the active parts of this living inner layer of the skin. Then, on top of the dermis, lies the epidermis – a thin outer layer without blood vessels and only a few nerve endings reaching into it. The epidermis is itself made up of layers. The first (inner) layer consists of fresh living skin cells which reproduce like all living cells and then pass into the next layer. Here the cells are starting to become drier and more leathery, and as they make their way up, layer by layer, to the outer surface of the skin, so they gradually dry out and die.

The dead top layer of the epidermis can take quite a few bangs and knocks before it flakes off for good. For this reason, many minor scratches never reach the living cells below; all the damage is revealed in a thin white line across the skin where the dead cells have been lifted. But if the scratch goes a little deeper, then it can reach beyond the epidermis to the tiny blood vessels in the dermis, perhaps rupturing one or two, so that the scratch shows up red or even bleeds slightly. If the skin is actually cut, then the clotting ability of the blood, combined with the readiness of the skin cells in the epidermis to migrate sideways and seal the gap, soon heals the wound.

CROSS-SECTION THROUGH THE SKIN

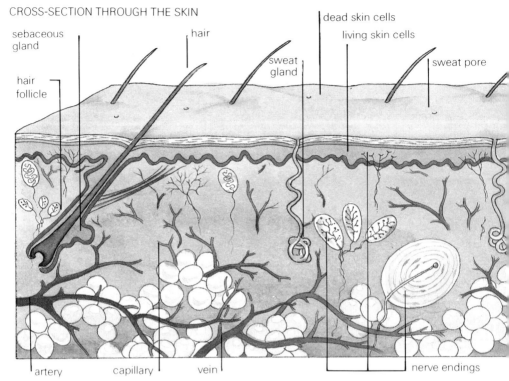

sebaceous gland

hair

dead skin cells

living skin cells

hair follicle

sweat gland

sweat pore

artery

capillary

vein

nerve endings

The tiny blood vessels (or capillaries) in the skin have a crucial role to play in keeping the body at an even temperature, whatever climate we find ourselves in. The nerve endings detect the outside temperature, and if we need to cool down, messages are sent to the brain to pump as much blood as possible to the capillaries at the surface, so that a large quantity of blood can be cooled by the air around us. If the air is too warm to allow the blood to cool quickly enough, then the skin opens up its sweat glands, allowing water out onto the surface, where it can evaporate. The process of evaporation cools the skin, helping to cool the blood in the capillaries. And the same reactions are triggered from inside the body if we are exercising vigorously and start to overheat.

When our bodies are too cold, the

The complex world of the human skin. The diagram (above) shows details which are hard to see in the real cross-section (top right) where the hair roots stand out (magnified 200 times).

You can see a wound healing in the cross-section opposite.

reverse happens. The capillaries are practically shut down, so that our blood stays deeper inside our bodies, kept warm by the insulating layer of fat in the dermis. The sweat glands remain tightly shut, so no evaporation takes place; and our skin comes out in goose pimples. Each little raised dot of skin in fact contains a tiny hair; and the goose-pimpling reaction makes that hair stand on end. Between the upright hairs a layer of air is trapped all

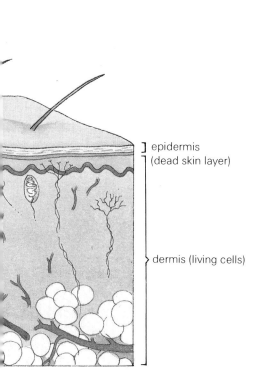

epidermis
(dead skin layer)

dermis (living cells)

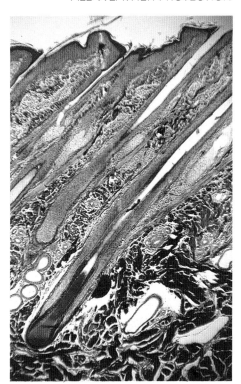

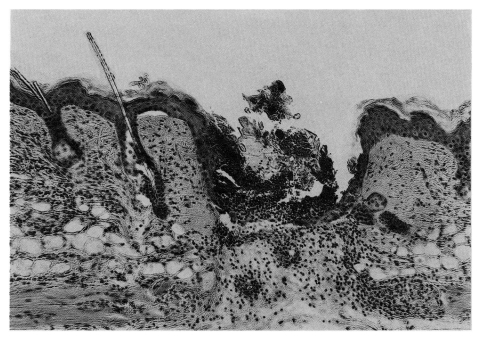

around the body; and as air is a poor con-ductor of heat, this also improves the body's insulation.

Naturally, these hairs are yet another vital part of the total all-weather protec-tion system. When we are very warm and the hairs are lying down flat, air can pass directly over the skin, without being trapped against it, and so heat from the body is carried away. With so many different regulators to adjust, the skin is remarkably efficient at maintaining a constant body temperature, whatever we are doing and in whatever surrounding temperature.

If it all sounds too good to be true, there is a drawback. It is not only temperature changes which can activate this system; emotional reactions do so as well. You can have sweaty hands from feeling anxious, and it is so hard to control the reaction that sensitive sweat detectors can tell when your anxiety level goes up even minimally, for instance every time you tell a lie. Polygraphs (or lie detectors) work in part by monitoring this sweat reaction. And of course your skin doesn't only red-den when you are too hot. Embarrass-ment causes the same sort of blushing, so your real feelings are almost impossible to hide. Your skin may give you excellent pro-tection, but it does tend to give you away as well!

GETTING TO GRIPS WITH THINGS

Our hands can reveal the most profound and sensitive emotions, either through brush strokes on a canvas, or a delicate touch on the strings or stops of a musical instrument. They can also wrestle with alligators and climb the sheer face of the Matterhorn, caress a lover and portray the pure poetry of a ballerina's dance. And yet, for all this wondrous ability, our hands in themselves are little more than a collection of skin, nerves and bone, held together by a few tiny muscles and tendons. They are like marionettes, cleverly strung together but lifeless, relying entirely on remote control before the genius of Picasso, Yehudi Menuhin or Margot Fonteyn can flow from their fingertips.

But even if we have to acknowledge the all-important role of the powerful muscles in our forearms, and the essential control of the brain, we can still find some marvellous craftsmanship and engineering in the way our hands get to grips with things. Pick up something about as heavy as a large bottle of lemonade in one hand, and look closely at your fingertips, which will be white where the pressure of your grip has squeezed the blood from the capillaries. This is because the soft flesh of each fingertip is moulded to take the shape of the surface being gripped, and then compressed into a firm clamping pad by being pushed back hard against the fingernail. In addition, the tiny ridges that give us our fingerprints, and the minute amounts of sweat we excrete between them, combine to help ensure that our grip stays firm and does not slip. The fingerprints we leave behind for the detectives to discover are in fact tiny lines of moisture which enable the spaces between the whorls and ridges of the fingertip to become little suction pads. When delicately dusted, they show up as the unique trademark of whoever gripped the bottle.

Notice, also, the positioning of the fingers. Without you being aware of it, they have spread themselves out into a fan arrangement, with the four longer fingers all pressing one way and the thumb pressing in the opposite direction. Because the thumb 'opposes' the other fingers like this, insurers acknowledge that it is the most vital part of the hand. You can grip most things reasonably easily without one, two, or even three of the other four fingers making up one half of the pincer grip. But the other half of the pincer consists of the thumb alone.

The power for this pincer grip, and for most of our hand movements, comes from big muscles in the forearm. Roll up your

77

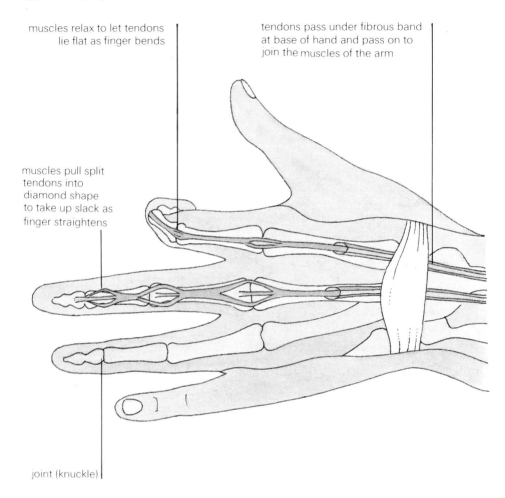

muscles relax to let tendons
lie flat as finger bends

tendons pass under fibrous band
at base of hand and pass on to
join the muscles of the arm

muscles pull split
tendons into
diamond shape
to take up slack as
finger straightens

joint (knuckle)

sleeve, clench and unclench your fist while turning the hand from side to side, and you should be able to see the muscles in action – contracting and relaxing in turn. If you are in any doubt, lightly grip the forearm with your other hand; you will then quite easily feel the muscles at work. As these muscles contract, they pull on the 'marionette strings' which operate the hand. These strong flexible tissues, called tendons, run into the hand under a 'bridge' of fibrous tissue which holds them in as they go past the wrist. They then fan out amongst the fat, muscle, blood ves-

In this simplified diagram you can clearly see how the splits in the tendons on a straightened finger are pulled open at the knuckles, and how on a bent finger they lie closed together.

sels, nerves and numerous cleverly inter-linked bones of the hand itself. And each tendon finishes up joined to the one part of the hand it will help to move. We can appreciate the skilful arrangement of the entire network of tendons if we explore the workings of just one finger.

In each finger there are two joints, or

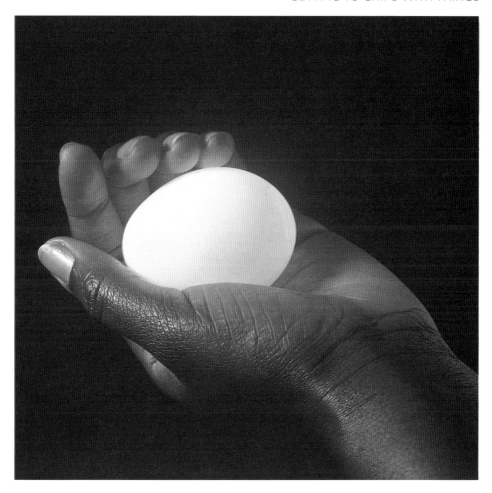

Close your fingers around an egg and think about how sensitive your nerve endings need to be so that you grip the egg but do not crush it.

knuckles if you like. On the inside of the hand, one long tendon runs all the way up to the bone above the top joint, ready to bend that bit of the finger inwards. As it passes the joint below, it divides rather cleverly, leaving a gap through which a second tendon can pass. This is attached to the bone just above that joint, so that the top two sections of the finger can be pulled inwards. By operating both tendons at once, the whole finger can be curled round, perhaps to grip something. Or, if all four fingers of an empty hand are curled in this way at the same time, we can make a fist.

Tendons running along the tops of the fingers are then pulled by muscles in the forearm to open the hand by pulling the fingers out straight again. If you run a length of sticky tape around the outside curve of a clenched finger and onto the back of the hand, you will be following the

79

kind of path one of these tendons takes. Now straighten the finger, and you will notice that the tape has to ruckle up, because the distance around a clenched finger is obviously much greater than the distance along the back of a straightened one. The contracted muscle in the forearm will 'reel in' some of this length as it straightens the finger, but it cannot manage all of it. So an ingenious arrangement in the finger itself 'absorbs' the extra bit of tendon. The tendon is in fact split where it runs over the knuckle at the bottom of the finger, and tiny muscles on either side of the knuckle pull one half of the split tendon away from the central line of the finger and down round the side of it.

If you cut yourself a strip of paper and put a slit down the middle of it, like a buttonhole, you can see how well it works. Notice how far apart the ends of the strip are when it is lying flat; then pick it up by the middle of the two sides, and open the slit by pulling the two sides apart – exactly as the muscles do to the split finger tendon. Now look and see how much closer the two ends of the strip are to each other.

For the brain to make the most of this clever engineering, it has to receive a tremendous amount of information about what is going on when our hands are in contact with something. The force we need to grip and lift a sack of coal will be very different from that needed to pick up an egg without breaking it. We also need to know if something is too hot or cold for us to handle, whether it has sharp edges which will cut us, and so on. Not surprisingly, our fingertips need a huge number of sensitive nerve endings to take in all this information. Shut your eyes and get a friend to touch your fingertip with two pins held so close together that you cannot tell whether there are one or two points touching you. Then ask your friend to touch you again, with the points a fraction of a millimetre further apart, and keep repeating this until you can feel two distinct points.

Remember how far apart the points are, and then do the experiment all over again on your forearm. You will be amazed at the difference! The reason the points are so far apart before you can detect both of them on your forearm is that there are far fewer nerve endings there. And so the forearm is not as sensitive as the much tinier fingertips. A good job too – imagine having to design a piano on which Chopin could be played with the forearms!

SORTING OUT THE BOYS FROM THE GIRLS

The tour of our citadel is barely half completed, yet there are surprisingly few new things left for us to see, despite the fact that we have not even noticed whether we are in a male or a female citadel. As we retrace our steps from the fingertips, along the arms and back into the main trunk of the body, we are fairly familiar with much of what we see. After all, both our arms have the same sort of biological hinge and lever arrangements – bones covered with muscles, blood vessels and nerves. And inside the trunk, we have already seen the heart – a four-chambered mass of muscle, with a clever system of valves, which keeps the blood moving all round the body. So we can hurry on, getting down to just above waist level before we come to anything new.

There we will discover the large smooth-surfaced liver, an essential factory for extracting certain food chemicals from the blood, reshaping and changing some of them, and controlling the quantities to be distributed around the body. Inside the tight spongy corridors of the liver, the factory's 'employees' (more of those chemicals called enzymes) take over where the enzymes in the gut left off. For instance, they quite happily allow enough of the protein in the blood to flow on through the liver for distribution to all parts of the body. But if you have eaten more protein than you need, then most of the excess is converted by the enzymes into storable carbohydrates instead of being rejected as waste. The liver also breaks down other products in the blood (such as dead red blood cells and alcohol), retaining and storing anything useful and sending the disposable waste products to the kidneys via the bloodstream.

Our two kidneys lie towards the back of the body, behind the intestines; and they act as filters, removing waste products from the blood through a series of tiny sieve-like pockets into which the blood is pumped, and out of which it can only trickle away slowly. The pressure of the blood building up in the sieves pushes small waste molecules through the tiny holes in the sieves; larger molecules, such as the blood cells and useful foods, cannot get out. The cleansed blood continues on its way round the body, while the squeezed-out waste products, carried in a little water which was squeezed out with them, are sent to the bladder as urine. There it is stored until we can conveniently get rid of it.

So all that we have yet to explore in the lower cavity of the trunk, surrounded by the coiled pipework of the intestines, are the sex organs. You might think that

81

These simplified diagrams give a good idea of how either male or female sex organs develop from the same part of an embryo. Before the sex of the baby has been determined, the gonads will develop (opposite). They can then be triggered to develop into a male (below, left) or remain female (below, right). The development of the womb and ovaries is not shown.

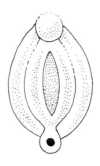

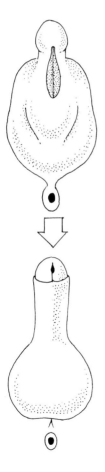

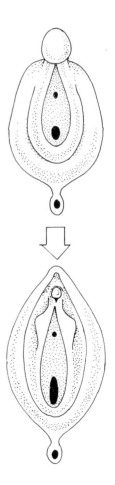

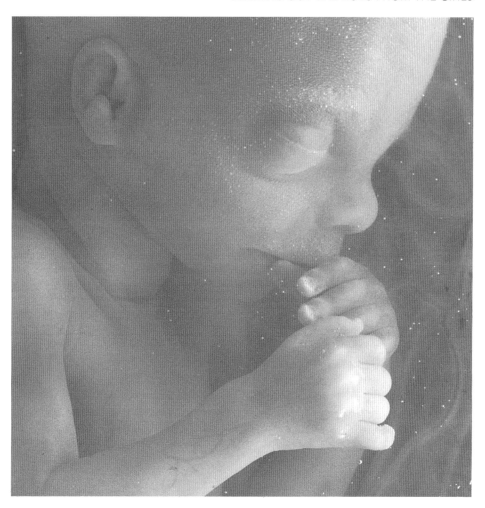

people are radically different in this area, depending on whether they are male or female; but in fact the male and female sex organs, both internal and external, develop from an identical set of primitive organs, or gonads. For the first few weeks after conception, the baby developing in its mother's womb is neither male nor female. It has no sex organs apart from the gonads, and they could develop into either male or female sex organs. If the gonads become ovaries, then a large muscular bag (the womb or uterus) devel-

This baby is less than halfway through its development in the womb, but 16 weeks after conception every tiny feature can be clearly seen.

ops between them, opening out into the female vagina. If the gonads become testes, no uterus develops, but a male penis evolves, and the testes eventually descend into sacs of skin below it. This leaves a space in the male body where the female uterus is located.

Rather than go into the well-known

83

details of how males and females get their enjoyable act together and sometimes reproduce, it might be more interesting to find out how this anatomical layout gave rise to a bizarre theory in the mid-1980s. Some scientists quite seriously claimed that it might be technically possible for a male to allow a baby to develop inside his body for the full term of pregnancy, rather than have the mother carry the baby in the normal way.

The idea arose largely because of the extraordinary experience of a New Zealand woman, Margaret Martin, who had her uterus surgically removed, leaving her with no womb for a baby to develop in. Yet, amazingly, she began to experience all the symptoms of pregnancy. Eventually, scans revealed that there was a baby growing inside her abdomen. And, some months later, it was successfully delivered during an operation rather like a caesarean section, in which the mother was carefully cut open and the baby lifted out.

What must have happened was that just prior to her hysterectomy, when the uterus was removed, an egg was produced in Mrs Martin's ovaries. The egg was fertilised by her husband's sperm, and then escaped into the abdomen as the womb was removed. There it was able to implant on the outside wall of the large intestine, where the tissues, having a rich blood supply, are not totally dissimilar to those lining the womb. The baby managed to thrive in this unusual environment until the successful delivery operation gave Mrs Martin a healthy baby daughter. If it all worked out well for her, the scientists thought, why not fertilise an egg in the laboratory, and then put this test-tube baby into the father's abdomen, where it could grow on the wall of the large intestine until it was developed enough to be removed in an operating theatre?

However, when doctors and other scientists studied the proposal carefully, most of them eventually concluded that it was far too risky and difficult. To start with, they thought the only way to get the fertilised egg to embed itself on the wall of the large intestine would be to let it float around the abdomen until it found a resting place. This meant that it could end up on a kidney or the liver, or some vital blood vessel, which could seriously interfere with any of those organs, and even prove fatal. More likely, in any case, the egg would never implant successfully, and would simply die before it had even begun to develop. The fact that Mrs Martin's case was so extraordinary suggests that her successful outcome is the exception rather than the rule, and so-called male pregnancy is really not a practical proposition.

Nevertheless, the whole fascinating episode reminds us just how similar males and females are. Our entire sexuality depends on how two tiny gonads develop just 6 weeks after conception; and apart from our sex organs, our bodies are virtually interchangeable. Not as fundamental a difference as some people of both sexes would prefer there to be!

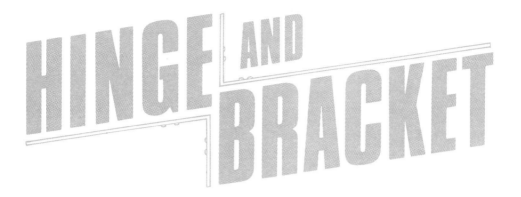

HINGE AND BRACKET

Once past the sex organs and into the legs, we are soon in very familiar territory. At first sight, the legs seem to follow the same design as our arms – a set of long bones which can bend and twist with the help of muscles all around them. Even the feet at the end of them are remarkably similar to our hands.

This should not be too surprising. After all, most other animals do not have one pair of limbs which differs from the other. We happily refer to all four of their limbs as 'legs'. They walk, grip and fight with all four, and only rarely bare their underbellies to the world by standing upright on two limbs. Even the apes spend most of their time slouching, crouching or scurrying on all fours. In contrast, we have evolved so that we stand proudly erect from barely a year old; and we walk, run and jump with only two limbs, leaving our other two to specialise in holding and manipulating.

This explains some of the obvious differences between arms and legs, hands and feet. Our fingers are longer and more versatile than our toes. And our thigh muscles are bigger and more powerful than our upper arm muscles, having to support the weight of the whole body all the time, as well as move our legs. Clearly, the bones in our arms and legs are slightly different in

size and shape according to the specialist tasks of each limb. So too are the joints; our wrists, for instance, are looser and more flexible than our ankles, to give us the dexterity we demand of our hands. At the same time, our ankles need to be firmer, in order to help us stay upright while balancing the whole weight of our bodies on remarkably small areas: the flat foot as we stand, the balls of our feet as we walk and run, and even the few square centimetres at the tips of our toes as we peer over high fences or dance on our pointes.

As specialist as they are, all our joints rely on the same basic tissues to hinge and bracket our hands and feet to our lower limbs, our upper limbs to these lower ones, and our limbs to our trunk. And so a quick look at one joint, such as the knee, will soon reveal not only how cleverly all our joints are made, but also how they are each adapted to the very specific tasks required of them.

Think of parachutists and high-jumpers. Both depend enormously on having effective knees. When parachutists hit the ground, they will be putting forces up to 25 times their own weight through their knees. So a knee has to be strong and shock-absorbent. When high-jumpers run up, take off, and twist and rotate their bodies as they lift themselves over the bar, they make quite different demands on their knees. They need the flexible hinge quality to allow for a fluent run-up and a firm, momentary locking ability to make the leg stiff as they take off, in order to use the power of the spring to lift the whole body off the ground. Then, almost instantly, they need to rotate and twist the knee to allow the upper torso to change direction from that of the run-up and take-off, ahead of the lower legs, as it flattens itself out and clears the bar.

You can easily observe these abilities in your own knee. While seated with your legs together but not crossed, raise one foot off the floor. Keeping the knee bent and swinging the lower leg backwards and forwards, you will of course see the basic hinging of the knee. But if you now hold your knee, with both hands pressing gently into the knee just below the knee-cap and to each side of it, you will feel its rotation ability. Simply turn your foot from side to side, keeping your ankle stiff, and your hands should feel the bones moving in the lower half of the knee.

Next, unless you are reading this in a train and already getting curious looks, stretch your leg straight out. As you rotate your foot now, you cannot feel those bones moving. Instead, your whole leg is rotating, because the knee has locked in a straightened position. This gives the leg enormous strength, so that you can stand up and bear weight for ages without unduly tiring your muscles. Try standing up now, with your legs bent and the knees in the unlocked position. Apart from looking strangely weak-kneed, you will soon find your thigh muscles aching, longing for you to stand up straight, lock your knees and give them a rest!

The reason for all these abilities is the

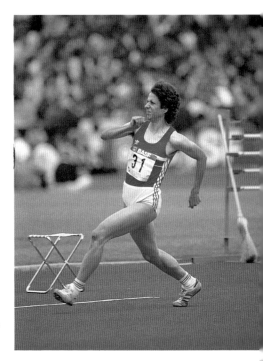

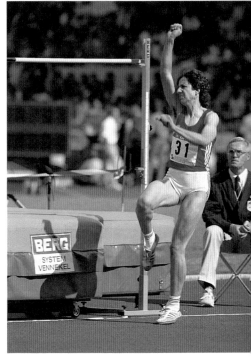

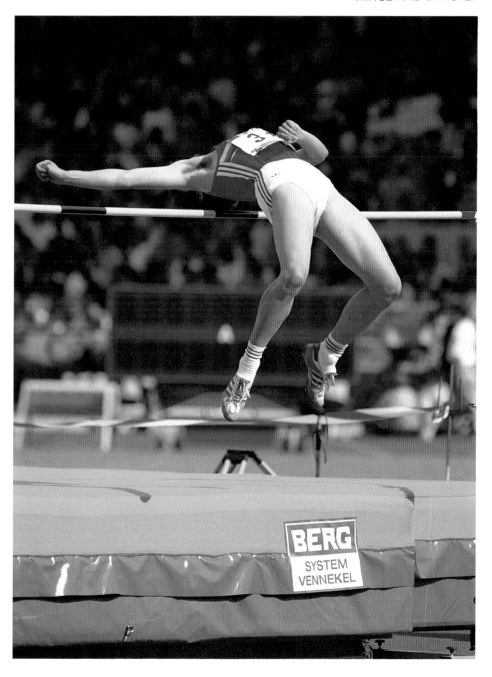

The high-jumper's run-up (top left) makes a very different demand on the knee joint from the lift-off (opposite) and the rotation and lay back over the bar (above).

87

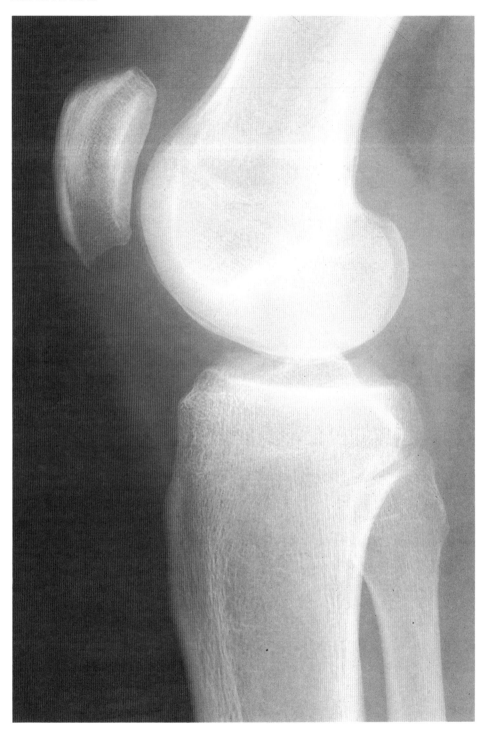

knee's stunningly simple and effective design. There are no special complex parts – just precisely shaped ends to the bones which meet at the knee. They are tied together with tough, elastic tissues called ligaments, which are cunningly threaded like laces in a shoe to hold everything in exactly the right position for whatever demand we are placing on the knee. Some of them run straight down the outsides of the bones being joined; and others cross over each other, running through the middle of the joint. Then, just to make everything work smoothly, the ends of the bones are covered in a coating of cartilage – a bit like the non-stick surface on a frying pan. This allows for some of the required shock absorbency, as well as ensuring that the hinge does not stick. Add a kneecap – a tiny pad of bone to protect the knee, particularly when we kneel down – and you have the complete joint.

The key to it all is the way in which the ends of the two main bones which meet at the knee slot together. They fit rather like a loosely cut dovetail joint when the leg is straight, so that one bone cannot turn or twist without turning the other. In this way the knee is locked. This means that, when the knee bends, it cannot simply open and close like a hinge. As we bend it, the upper or thigh bone slides forward slightly over the end of the lower leg bone, separating the two halves of the dovetail. This allows the knee to unlock and the bones to turn separately from each other, moving smoothly as one cartilage-covered surface slides on the other. Only the strength of the ligaments and muscles now holds

An X-ray reveals the clever shape of the ends of the bones which create the knee, but not the ligaments which hold them together.

the knee together, but the shape of the ends of the bones still restricts the amount each bone can move relative to the other. After all, if we were able to turn our lower legs right round in a complete circle, we could spin them round and round. This would have the effect of twisting up the ligaments, rather like winding up the propeller on a model aeroplane. Just as this twists up the rubber bands which drive the aeroplane, so such spinning of the lower leg would eventually strain, wear out and tear the ligaments.

All our joints, not only the knee, rely on a similar arrangement. And you can see this most easily, ironically enough, in an abnormal situation. Some people are born with unusually long and flexible ligaments, and they can allow their bones to stretch apart so much that they move beyond the point where the shape of the bones restricts the movement of the joints. We call such people 'double-jointed' and they sometimes perform on the stage as contortionists. The point is that all their joints are loose, not just the knees, so you can see by their abnormal movements just where the limits on our more normal movement are imposed by the shape of the ends of our bones.

In the end, though, the stability of any joint depends mostly on the muscles which surround it. Otherwise double-jointed people would not be able to control their knees sufficiently to stand upright. This is also why professional footballers, and other athletes who might easily damage their knees, have to build up their quadriceps muscles to hold them firmly. But if, despite everything, the ligaments do get torn, then healing can be a lengthy process; and often the ligaments simply do not reattach to the bones and the knee is left permanently weakened. In some cases, strips of stretchy artificial fibres like Dacron are used as crude artificial ligaments. They are surgically attached to the relevant points in the bones, often by being pulled through holes specially drilled into them, and then threaded through the knee in place of the real ligaments. It works surprisingly well; international sports stars have gone on playing at the top of their sports with this kind of repair to their knees.

But if the fundamental design of the joint is damaged, then repairs are not nearly so easy. Cartilage damage, and any subsequent wear and tear on the bones, will spoil the clever sliding, locking and unlocking mechanism provided by the carefully designed shape of the ends of our bones. Apart from sports injuries or sudden accidents, this damage is most commonly caused by the gradual progression of arthritis in the joint. In severe cases, artificial knees have to be surgically inserted to give the patient a reasonable degree of movement. Recently, they have even tried transplanting whole knees from one person to another, by cutting off the ends of the diseased bones and grafting into their place the completely joined ends of the healthy bones from a dead person. And this complex operation is necessary all because of the slightest of changes to the dips and hollows, rises and falls of the ends of our bones. It all goes to show that even the cleverest architects and designers are no match for evolution when it comes to human hinges and brackets.

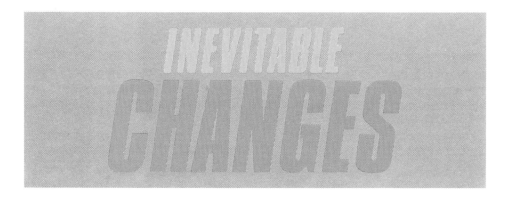

INEVITABLE CHANGES

Now that we have finally visited every corner of our citadel, we ought to be able to reflect on how old it is, and what sort of condition it is in. The passing of the days leaves its mark on our bodies as much as it does on any other thriving community. From the moment of conception we are constantly changing, undergoing sudden and radical changes, as well as the continual, slow changes built into our bodies from the outset. In a real citadel we would see these changes as the colour of the stone walls gradually darkening with the ravages of the climate, or imperceptibly wearing away until they were no longer able to go on serving their purpose. We would also see, from time to time, the sudden changes – the busy building of new roads or ramparts as the citizens redesigned their whole citadel to take account of new challenges as each new era dawned. If we look closely at our bodies over their lifetime we will see exactly the same kind of changes taking place.

The first dramatic change takes place 6 weeks after conception, when the gonads become sex organs. As with all the other sudden changes that are to follow it, the triggering mechanism is the action of hormones. These are the special chemicals which make contact with another chemi-cal, deoxyribonucleic acid (better known as DNA), in our living cells. The DNA contains a complete set of instructions for building and developing every part of our body; but not all the DNA is 'switched on' at the same time. In fact most of it is 'switched off' at any one point in time, and for the DNA in the cell to be useful it needs to be triggered into specific actions at different times and in different parts of the body. This allows some cells to become part of our skin, for instance, while others become part of our bones, or muscles, or whatever; and then the cells specialise further, so that some skin cells can become part of the eye, others part of the ear, and so on.

Hormones flooding into a cell and making contact with the DNA can trigger one part of the DNA to 'switch on'; and this is what usually happens when our bodies undergo sudden and dramatic changes. If the cells in the gonads of an embryo are not flooded with testosterone (the male hormone), they will continue to develop into female sex organs; but if enough sections of DNA are 'switched on' by the testosterone, then the gonads will become male sex organs. The choice is pretty definite – a bit like tossing a coin when you end up with either heads or tails. In the same way, even though the degree of maleness or femaleness can vary, there is normally a strong tendency for the gonads to make the embryo physically completely female, or completely male. But in very rare cases, as if the tossed coin had come down on its edge somehow, the embryo develops some male and some female physical characteristics.

There are no more sudden changes like this until well after birth; but as soon as a baby is born we can see several ways in which gradual continuous change is taking place. Take the skin, for example. A baby's skin is very soft and elastic; and even though it will need a few folds to allow the baby room to bend and stretch, none of those folds leaves a tell-tale line or wrinkle, such as we see in an older person. It is something we are all aware of. Think how many times, after a certain age, we peer into the mirror to see if the lines round our eyes are giving away how old we are!

Our skin cells are supported on a latticework of rubbery collagen. This collagen gradually gets less elastic and the latticework becomes more sagging and stretched. Eventually it loses so much of its resilience that the skin is unable to stay stretched tight and begins to wrinkle and fold in on itself, causing the wrinkles which appear around our face, limbs or trunk. Some people are so sensitive about aging that they desperately try to cover up their wrinkles; but there is no way of reversing the process, whatever cosmetic manufacturers might have you believe. In any case, wrinkles often produce characterful faces which some of us find more attractive than their smooth, elastic, younger versions!

Gradual changes, like the weakening of the collagen in the skin, are taking place all the time all over our bodies. Our eyes eventually take longer to change their focus, our bones become less flexible and more brittle, and so on. These are the inevitable changes of aging, built into our bodies from the very start. It seems as if they are important components in a system which ensures that we will eventually wear out and die at some fixed point in time, unless some untimely infection or disaster has cut us off earlier. Because we all see ourselves at the centre of our lives, it is perhaps not surprising if we regard the inevitability of our death as a tragedy. But in a broader context, our mortality is important. If we did not change, reproduce and die, apart from rapidly crowding out the planet, our species could not adapt to the changing world about us. We have evolved so that, over the centuries, only those people inheriting what are currently the best characteristics for the preservation of the human race will be able to survive and pass on their DNA to their children, and on to future generations. So the aging process is a vital part of human life, allowing for death and replacement to optimise the chances for the long-term survival of the human race.

In order to reproduce and create the next generation, our bodies need to go through the second of life's sudden changes, puberty. Boys become men and girls become women because of more hormones being released to 'switch on' the DNA in specific cells. Interestingly, the male hormone, testosterone, and the female hormone, oestrogen, are both released in male *and* female bodies. Besides altering the male larynx so that the voice 'breaks', and altering the size and shape of the male penis and testes while making the male able to produce sperm, the testosterone in males triggers

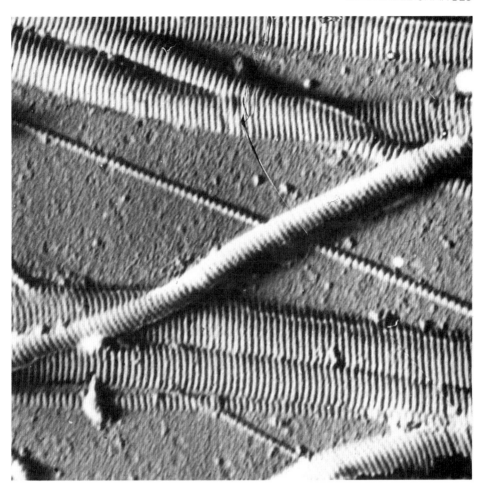

These rubbery, resilient, long strands of collagen will stretch, weaken, tear and tangle with age.

the growth of pubic and underarm hair. It triggers the same hair growth in women; but of course the development of their breasts and the changes in their sex organs so that they start releasing eggs and menstruating every month are all triggered by the female hormone, oestrogen.

While the male hormone produces the growth of body hair in females, the role of the oestrogen produced in males at

puberty is not so obvious. Both boys and girls have a rapid growth spurt at puberty; and this involves a third hormone, called growth hormone, being released in greater quantities than previously. This is triggered by both oestrogen and testosterone simultaneously, and the extra growth hormone in turn triggers an acceleration in the growth of our bones to their full size. So it is apparently only in this process that males make use of the extra female hormones being produced in their bodies. And, whether, we are male or female, with so many hormones rushing

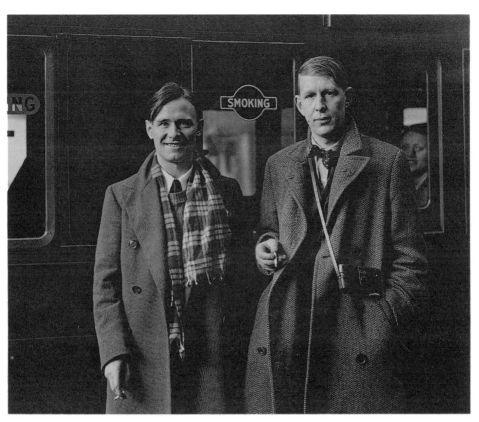

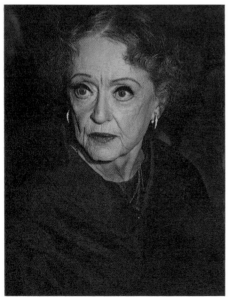

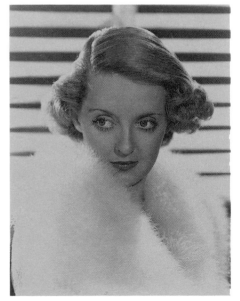

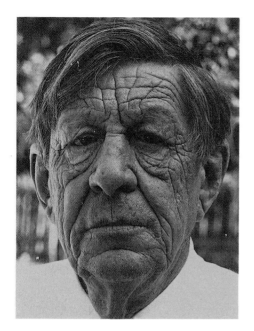

The effect of aging collagen on two famous faces; poet W. H. Auden (with Christopher Isherwood, opposite; and above) and Bette Davis. The older faces retain all the character of their unmistakable younger versions.

around the body, it is not surprising that most of us find puberty such a difficult and confusing time!

The final sudden change in life is the menopause. It is commonly assumed to be something which affects only women, but men do experience it too, though in a more gradual and less dramatic way. During the menopause, the production of the sex hormones is 'switched off'; and some people, especially women, may feel side effects, such as depression, which they can correct by taking hormone supplements. On the other hand, many women who cope positively with the menopause find advantages in being released from their regular menstrual cycle and its accompanying changes in mood.

In fact perhaps the most important thing about all the changes in our bodies is that they bring us new feelings, new challenges and new perspectives on life. If we were always the same, we would soon become bored, and we would not be able to make as much of our lives as we do. Even if changes seem unsettling to us at the time, they prepare us to cope with the next important stage ahead. Without childhood, we would not be free enough of other pressures to learn the basic skills of survival. Then puberty introduces the fertile years when our strongest drives are often towards home-building and raising the next generation. And finally the menopause releases us from these strenuous urges to ensure the survival of the human race; in effect, we lose the sex drives which urged us to reproduce ourselves. This has the advantage that we can begin to come to terms with our own mortality. As they reconcile themselves to the inevitability of their own eventual death, elderly people seem to find the prospect of it less frightening than they did in their fertile years. They often find contentment in enjoying the world for what it is, discovering a peace which younger people may not understand.

All this from the extraordinary putting together of some very common chemical elements. A cold statistical breakdown would reveal that we are mainly made up of carbon, hydrogen and oxygen, with small amounts of other elements thrown in for good measure. But this falls far short of revealing the amazing sophistication of the way we are built, and the way life surges through every living cell in our complex bustling citadels. We are naturally fascinated by ourselves; the wonders we discover when taking a magical mystery tour of our own flesh and blood give us every reason to marvel at what we find.

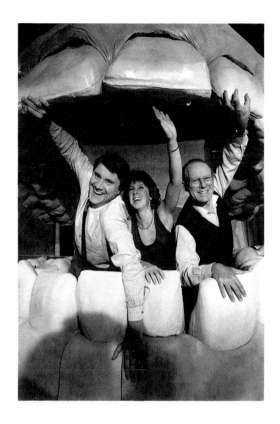

PHOTOGRAPHIC ACKNOWLEDGEMENTS

BBC HULTON PICTURE LIBRARY page 94 *top*; BIOPHOTO ASSOCIATES pages 44, 53 and 93; PROF. W. S. BULLOUGH page 75 *bottom*; CAMERA PRESS (P. Mitchell) page 95; BRUCE COLEMAN (Manfred Kage) page 29; COLORSPORT pages 86 *both* and 87; GEOSCIENCE FEATURES page 75 *top*; IMAGE BANK (Zao-Grimberg) page 45; KANEHARA SHUPPAN CO., TOKYO, from 'Tests for Colour-Blindness' by S. Ishihara, page 26; KOBAL COLLECTION page 94 *bottom left and right*; OSF (Carolina Biological Supply Co.) page 70–71; REX FEATURES pages 11, 66 and 67; ROYAL NATIONAL ORTHOPAEDIC HOSPITAL pages 72 *both* and 88; SCIENCE PHOTO LIBRARY pages 10 *both*, 16–17 (CNRI), 36 (CNRI), 37, 48 and 49 (*both* Prof. C. Ferlaud/CNRI), 51 (Dr K. F. R. Schiller), 57, 62 (Eric Grave) and 79 (Harry Nor-Hansen); TELEGRAPH COLOUR LIBRARY (S. J. Allen) page 83; ZEFA page 21.

The photographs on the front cover and page 96 were taken by the BBC.